Introduction
to
Toxicology

THIRD EDITION

Introduction
to
Toxicology

THIRD EDITION

John Timbrell

PROFESSOR OF BIOCHEMICAL TOXICOLOGY
DEPARTMENT OF PHARMACY
KING'S COLLEGE LONDON, UK

informa
healthcare

New York London

Informa Healthcare USA, Inc.
52 Vanderbilt Avenue
New York, NY 10017

10 9 8 7

International Standard Book Number-10: 0-4152-4763-2 (Softcover)
International Standard Book Number-13: 978-0-4152-4763-4 (Softcover)

Library of Congress Cataloging-in-Publication Data

Introduction to toxicology /
   John Timbrell. -- 3rd ed.
      p. ; cm.
   Includes bibliographical references and index.
   ISBN-13: 978-0-4152-4763-4 (Softcover : alk. paper)
   ISBN-10: 0-4152-4763-2 (Softcover : alk. paper)
   1. Toxicology. I. Title.
   [DNLM: 1. Toxicology. 2. Poisoning.
3. Poisons. QV 600 T583i 2002]

RA1211.T56 2002
615.9--dc21   2001053173

Visit the Informa Web site at
www.informa.com

and the Informa Healthcare Web site at
www.informahealthcare.com

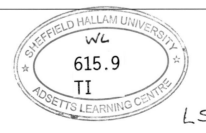

Contents

Preface to the first edition

There is an ever increasing use of chemicals in modern society and, because of this, toxicology is becoming an increasingly important subject. Taught courses are now available in different countries at various levels to educate young toxicologists. Currently, however, there are no introductory texts that are reasonable inexpensive, and that serve as an introduction to the subject for students with backgrounds in various disciplines. Thus, there are hardback textbooks, such as *Cassarett and Doull's Toxicology*, for dedicated toxicologists and various specialist texts for particular aspects of toxicology. The smaller textbooks that are available are generally biased towards one particular aspect or interpretation of toxicology, such as the biochemical, pathological, pharmacological or pharmacokinetic aspects. However, most of these are either too expensive or too specialist for the novice toxicologist, the undergraduate or the postgraduate who simply wishes to become familiar with the subject as a whole.

Toxicology is a multidisciplinary subject, which has a large and diffuse literature and it is developing rapidly. Bringing this information together is difficult and time consuming for the student. Consequently there is a need for a cohesive text at the introductory rather than more advanced level. These deficiencies in the market became clear to me whilst being involved in teaching first a Masters course and then a Bachelors degree course in toxicology.

This book, therefore, has arisen from my awareness of the need for an introductory text for myself and for my own students and its content is largely based upon the information I have amassed in the preparation of lectures for these same students. I am indebted to these students for being the foil for this preparation and also to various colleagues for their helpful comments.

London, 1988

Preface to the third edition

As with many areas of biomedical science, the study of toxicology has been influenced by fundamental changes in biochemistry and molecular biology and now by the newly emerging sciences of genomics, proteomics and metabonomics. These are having a major impact on the study and potentially an understanding of the interactions of chemicals with living sytems. Also new areas and types of interaction have emerged since the second edition of this book. Some of these, such as interactions with the peroxisome proliferator activated receptor, are now mentioned in this new edition. However, this book is primarily concerned with the basic underlying principles of toxicology at the introductory level and these remain largely unchanged. Therefore the *format* of the previous editions has been retained with specific examples used to illustrate these basic principles.

The major changes have been updating the existing text in relation to new knowledge or nomenclature and the inclusions of new examples. Thus there is now a much enlarged section on risk assessment and new sections on *in vitro* toxicology, on endocrine disrupters and on the treatment of posioning, for example. A number of specific case studies for particular chemicals or toxins have also been included.

This third edition now has chapter outlines and summaries and questions with answers, as teaching aids. For those requiring more extensive and detailed information there are a number of excellent reference texts which are listed in the bibliography at the end of each chapter.

The number of chemicals used in society will inevitably increase and consequently so will the risk of chemical exposure, even though the use and manufacture of chemicals may now be better regulated. Thus despite the recent regrettable closure, contraction or realignment of research institutions and courses specifically orientated towards toxicology in the UK, the subject of toxicology is no less important to our society. Therefore, scientists with a broad overview of toxicology will always be required as well as more specialized scientists such as molecular biologists. I hope that this book will help in that endeavour by stimulating an interest in toxicology.

As with previous editions, this third edition has benefited from my teaching activities at different levels and in many different places and countries for which I am grateful.

Finally, special thanks to Cathy for her specific help and support.

London, April 2001

CHAPTER 1

Introduction

Chapter outline

In this chapter you will learn about:

- The history of toxicology

- Types of toxic substance

- Types of exposure

- Selective toxicity

- The basic principles of the dose–response relationship

- Receptors

- ED_{50} and TD_{50}

- The therapeutic index

- Synergy and potentiation

- Threshold dose and NOAEL

Toxicology is the study of the harmful interactions between chemicals and biological systems. Man, the other animals, and the plants in the modern world are increasingly being exposed to chemicals of an enormous variety. These chemicals range from metals and inorganic chemicals to large complex organic molecules, yet they are all potentially toxic. The study of the pathological, biochemical and physiological effects of such substances is the fascinating brief of the toxicologist. Toxicology, like medicine, is a multidisciplinary subject which encompasses many areas. This makes it an absorbing and challenging area of research. The challenge of toxicology is to apply basic biochemical, chemical, pathological and physiological knowledge along with experimental observation to gain an understanding of why certain substances cause the disruption in a biological system which may lead to toxic effects.

Approximately 65 000 chemicals are currently produced in the USA and 500–1000 new chemicals are added each year. Because of this escalation in the numbers of chemicals to which our environment may be exposed (Figure 1.1), it has become increasingly important to have some knowledge of the toxic effects they may have and to attempt to measure and assess these effects.

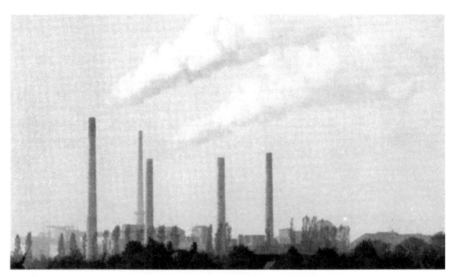

FIGURE 1.1 *Toxicology is concerned with the exposure of living systems in the environment to toxic substances from a variety of sources.*

In recent years, awareness of the problem of human and animal exposure to potentially toxic chemicals in our environment has grown. Perhaps one of the first to bring this to the attention of the public was Rachel Carson with her book ***Silent Spring***. This was a description of the devastating effects of pesticides on the flora and fauna of the North American environment. As discussed by Efron in her book ***The Apocalyptics, Cancer and the Big Lie*** (1984), Carson and certain later scientists probably exaggerated the dangers of chemicals, but her message was quite clear. Few would disagree that man should *be aware* of the synthetic chemicals to which the environment is exposed. Thus, toxicology has another dimension: the social, moral and legal aspects of exposure of populations to chemicals of unknown or uncertain hazard. Hazard and risk assessments and value judgements become important. The toxicologist is often asked to make such assessments and judgements. So toxicology has a very important role to play in modern society and consequently it is now growing rapidly as a new subject.

Historical aspects

Toxicology has been called the study of poisons, but this poses the question 'what is a poison?' Poisons can range from a naturally occurring plant alkaloid to a synthetic nerve gas. A poison is any substance which has a harmful effect on a living system; whether we regard a substance as a poison or not may depend on its use. For example, humans can protect themselves against the effects of harmful bacteria by killing them with antibiotics, such as **penicillin**; alternatively, humans can kill each other with the war gas **phosgene**. Both phosgene and penicillin, therefore, are poisons in the strictest sense of the word but we regard them entirely differently.

It is only recently that the study of poisons has become a truly scientific pursuit. In the past it was mainly a practical art utilized by murderers and assassins. Poison, as a subtle and silent weapon, has played an important part in human history.

Primitive man was aware of natural poisons from animals and plants and indeed used these on his weapons. The word toxicology is derived from *toxicon* – a poisonous substance into which arrow heads were dipped and *toxikos* – a bow. The study of poisons must have started by 1500 BC because the **Ebers Papyrus**, the earliest collection of medical records, contains many references and recipes for poisons. The ancient Egyptians were able to distil prussic acid from peach kernels, poisons such as arsenic, aconite and opium were also known to Hindu medicine as recorded in the **Vedas**, around 900 BC and the ancient Chinese used **aconite** as an arrow poison. **Hippocrates** in his writings (400 BC) showed that the ancient Greeks had a professional awareness of poisons and of the principles of toxicology, particularly with regard to the treatment of poisoning by influencing absorption. Poisoning was relatively common in ancient Greece so the study of poisons and the development of antidotes in particular was important. For example, **Nicander** of Colophon (185-135 BC), physician to Attalus, King of Bythnia, was allowed to experiment with poisons using condemned criminals as subjects. As a result of his studies he wrote a treatise on antidotes to poisonous reptiles and substances (Theriaca and Alexipharmica) and mentioned 22 specific poisons including **ceruse** (white lead), **litharge** (lead oxide), **aconite** (wolfsbane), **cantharides**, **conium** (hemlock), **hyoscyamus** (henbane) and **opium**. He recommended linseed tea to induce vomiting and sucking the venom from the bite of a venomous animal as treatments. Similarly, King **Mithridates** used criminals to search for antidotes to venom and poisonous substances and regularly protected himself with a mixture of 50 different antidotes (Mithridatum). Legend has it that he was unable to poison himself when suicide became necessary! The term **mithridatic** (meaning antidote) is derived from his name.

The first known law against poisoning was issued in Rome by Sulla in 82 BC to protect against careless dispensing. The Greek physician **Dioscorides** (AD 50) made a particularly significant contribution to toxicology by classifying poisons as animal, plant or mineral and recognizing the value of emetics in the treatment of poisoning. His treatise on Materia Medica was the major work on poisons for fifteen centuries.

So, the origins of toxicology lie in the use of poisons for murder, suicide and political assassination. It is well known for example that **Socrates** committed suicide by taking hemlock (Figure 1.2). There are many examples of poisons being used for nefarious purposes such as the poisoning of Claudius and his son Britannicus with **arsenic**. In the latter case, Nero employed a professional poisoner who put the arsenic into the water used to cool the soup and so avoided the taster. The prolific use of poisons in this way made it necessary for treatments to be devised and **Maimmonides** (1135–1204) wrote *Poisons and Their Antidotes* which detailed some of the treatments thought to be effective.

In the Middle Ages, especially in Italy, the art of poisoning for political ends developed into a cult. The **Borgias** were infamous during the fifteenth and sixteenth centuries. In seventeenth-century Italy, a woman by the name of Toffana prepared cosmetics containing arsenic (**Aqua Toffana**) which were used to remove unwanted rivals, husbands and enemies! Similarly **Catherine de Medici** prepared poisons and tested them on the poor and sick of France, noting all the clinical signs and symptoms.

One of the most important concepts in toxicology was espoused in the sixteenth century by a scientist by the name of **Paracelsus**. He was born Philippus Theophrastus Aureolus Bombastus von Hohenheim near Zurich in 1493 and was the son of a physician who was interested in chemistry and biology and was an

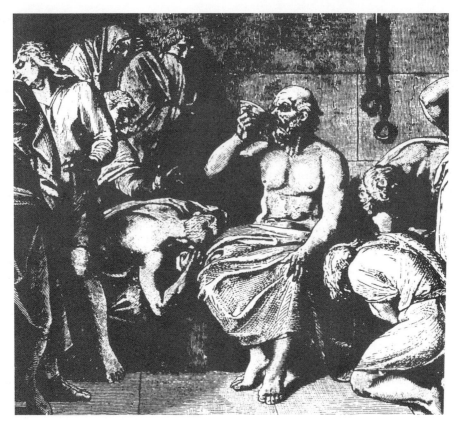

FIGURE 1.2 *Socrates drinking hemlock, the Athenian state poison. Reproduced with permission from the Mary Evans Picture Library, London.*

expert in occupational medicine. Paracelsus was a free thinker who disagreed with the dogma current at the time and espoused by Galen. Paracelsus thought observation was crucial and understood the importance of chemistry in medicine. He believed that 'like cures like', contrary to Galen who taught that diseases of a particular intensity would be cured by a medicine of opposite intensity. Consequently in the view of Paracelsus 'a poison in the body would be cured by a similar poison – but the dosage is very important'.

He advocated inorganic chemicals, such as salts, as treatments. These were believed to be too poisonous but he emphasized that the dose was very important. Paracelsus summarized this concept in the following famous phrase: 'All substances are poisons; there is none that is not a poison. The right dose differentiates a poison from a remedy.'

This concept is especially crucial to the safe use of drugs but also important for the safe handling of other chemicals (see below this chapter). It underlies the risk assessment of chemicals because from this relationship follows assessment of threshold doses and safe and non-toxic levels (see below Chapter 12). Even seemingly innocuous substances such as common salt could become poisonous under certain conditions. Paracelsus also believed that diseases were localized to particular organs and also that poisons would damage particular organs (target organs) something we now also know to be generally true.

His contribution to medicine and toxicology was enormous although not recognized until after his death in 1541.

Another significant figure in toxicology was **Orfila**, a Spanish physician (1787–1853) who recognized it as a separate discipline and contributed to forensic toxicology by devising means of detecting poisonous substances and therefore proving that poisoning had taken place. From then on toxicology began to develop in a more scientific manner and began to include the study of the mechanism of action of poisons. Indeed **Claude Bernard** (1813–1878) believed that the study of the effects of substances on biological systems could enhance the understanding of those systems. He identified the site of action of **curare** as either the nerve ending or the neuromuscular junction.

More recently, in 1945, Sir Rudolph **Peters** studied the mechanism of action of arsenical war gases and so was able to devise an effective antidote known as British Anti-Lewisite for the treatment of soldiers exposed to these gases. Other examples of toxic chemicals which have been studied at the mechanistic level with benefits for our understanding of basic biochemistry are cyanide and fluorocitrate. Cyanide inhibits the mitochondrial electron transport chain and fluorocitrate inhibits aconitase, one of the enzymes of the Krebs cycle.

Toxicology has now become much more than the use of poisons for nefarious purposes and the production of antidotes to them. The enormous and ever increasing number (65 000+) of man-made chemicals in the environment to which we may potentially be exposed has thrust toxicology into the limelight. It has also created the need for the organized study of toxic substances by the industries manufacturing them and for legislation to control them. This has in turn resulted in the establishment of government regulatory agencies to implement the resulting legislation.

Some of the industrial disasters which have occurred in recent times have highlighted the need for knowledge of the toxicity of compounds used in industry as well as for drugs and food additives. This knowledge is essential for the development of effective and rapid treatment of the toxic effects, just as it is essential for the treatment of overdoses and accidental poisonings. For example, one of the worst industrial disasters occurred at **Bhopal** in India in 1984 where a factory manufacturing the insecticide carbaryl leaked a large amount of the extremely noxious compound **methyl isocyanate** (Figure 1.3). Little was known of the toxicity of this compound and consequently treatment of the victims was uncertain and possibly inadequate.

Another major reason for testing chemicals in toxicity and other studies is so that they may be classified according to hazard such as toxic, explosive or flammable. This will then enable decisions to be made about marketing and labelling. So we are exposed to toxic or potentially toxic compounds in many ways in our daily lives and toxicology is clearly a subject of great importance in society. This becomes apparent when we look at the types of poisons and the ways in which we are exposed to them. Indeed, the categories cover virtually all the chemicals one might expect to encounter in the environment. After consideration of this one might well ask '*are all chemicals toxic?*' The following phrase perhaps provides an answer: '*there are no safe chemicals, only safe ways of using them.*'

Types of toxic substance

Toxic substances fall into several classes in relation to the way man is exposed to them: drugs, food additives, pesticides, industrial chemicals,

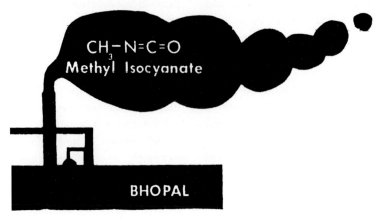

Bhopal: disaster seeking an antidote

$$CH_3 - N = C = O$$
Methyl Isocyanate

BHOPAL

FIGURE 1.3 *A headline reminds us that a year after the disaster in Bhopal, India, in which thousands were killed and injured by the toxic chemical methyl isocyanate accidentally released from a chemical plant, there is no cure or antidote. Headline from* **The Sunday Times**, *1 December 1985, with permission.*

environmental pollutants, natural toxins and household poisons. Each of these categories will be discussed in more detail in later chapters but they will be briefly introduced here.

DRUGS

Most people in the Western world consume drugs of one sort or another throughout their lives. Drugs, however, have usually been designed to be highly potent in biological systems and consequently many are potentially toxic. Drug toxicity may be due either to an overdose or it may be a rare and unusual adverse effect, and examples of both of these will be considered in detail in Chapter 5.

Drugs vary enormously in chemical structure and possess a wide variety of biological activities. They are probably the only foreign substances of known biological activity that man ingests intentionally. Included in this category are alcohol and the active principles in cigarettes, both of which are used because of their

biological activity and both, of course, have toxic properties. Drugs used in veterinary practice must also be considered here (and in the next section) as humans may consume meat from or other food derived from animals treated with these drugs.

FOOD ADDITIVES

This is the second category of foreign substances which are directly ingested. However, food additives are usually of low biological activity. Many different additives are now added to food to alter the flavour or colour, prevent spoilage, or in some other way change the nature of the foodstuff. There are also many potentially toxic substances which may be regarded as contaminants occurring naturally in food, resulting from cooking, or from other contamination, and specific examples will be discussed in a later chapter. Veterinary drugs and their breakdown products may also be found in foodstuffs as indicated above. Most of these substances, both natural and artificial, may be present in food in very small amounts but for the majority little is known of their long-term toxicity. In many cases they are ingested daily for perhaps a lifetime and the numbers of people exposed is very large. Although reliable data are still scarce, there certainly seems to be evidence that at least some additives may be associated with adverse effects. Public awareness of this has now begun to influence the preparation and manufacture of food such that additive free foods are appearing on supermarket shelves.

INDUSTRIAL CHEMICALS

Industrial chemicals may contribute to environmental pollution (considered next), and they may be a direct hazard in the workplace where they are used, formulated or manufactured. There is a huge range of chemical types and many different industries may involve the use or manufacture of hazardous chemicals. In the broadest sense industrial exposure might include exposure to the solvents used in photocopiers and typists' correction fluid. Although in general exposure is controlled by law, often by the setting of control limits, realistic levels may still prove to be hazardous in the long term and acute exposure due to accidents will always occur. The long development time of diseases such as cancer often makes it difficult to determine the cause until sufficient of the workforce have presented with the disease for the association with the toxic compound to be made.

ENVIRONMENTAL POLLUTANTS

The main sources of pollution are industrial processes and the deliberate release into the environment of substances such as pesticides. The most visible pollutant, but perhaps not the most significant, is smoke from power stations and factories. Factories may also produce and emit more potent substances in smaller quantities although the level of these is generally controlled. Environmental pollutants may be released into the air, river or sea water or dumped onto land. Car exhaust fumes with several known toxic constituents constitute a major source of pollution.

Pesticides are deliberately sprayed onto crops or agricultural land with the potential for exposure either via the crop itself or through contamination of drinking water or air. With pesticides a major problem is persistence in the environment and an increase in concentration during passage through the food chain.

NATURAL TOXINS

Many plants and animals produce toxic substances for both defensive and offensive purposes. Natural toxins of animal, plant and bacterial origin comprise a wide variety of chemical types, cause a variety of toxic effects and are a significant cause of human poisonings. The concept currently expounded by some individuals that '*natural is safe*' is in many cases very far from the truth and some of the most toxic substances known to man are of natural origin. Natural toxins may feature in poisoning via contamination in food, by accidental ingestion of poisonous plants or animals, and by stinging and biting.

HOUSEHOLD POISONS

These may include some of the substances in the other categories such as pesticides, drugs and solvents. Exposure to these types of compounds is usually acute rather than chronic. Many of the household substances used for cleaning are irritants and some are corrosive.

Consequently, they may cause severe skin and eye lesions to humans if they are exposed. If swallowed in significant quantities or if highly concentrated solutions are ingested, some household materials such as bleach and caustic soda can cause severe tissue damage to the oesophagus and stomach. Some of the drugs and pesticides which are widely available and consequently often found in the home are also very toxic. For example, the herbicide paraquat and the drug paracetamol are both toxic and have both contributed significantly to human poisoning deaths.

Types of exposure

In some cases the means of exposure is determined by the nature of the toxic substance. For example, gases and vapours lead to inhalation exposure whereas liquids give rise to problems associated with skin contact. Many industrial chemicals are often associated with chronic effects due to long-term exposure whereas household substances are usually involved in acute poisoning following a single episode of accidental exposure.

The types of exposure will be briefly discussed at this introductory stage but will be discussed again more fully in later chapters.

INTENTIONAL INGESTION

Drugs and food additives are taken in by many millions of people every day, in some cases for long periods of time. The exposure to these compounds, especially repeated or chronic exposure, may be associated with adverse responses such as allergic reactions. Alcohol and cigarettes are used by many people, often on a long-term basis, and these may lead to chronic toxic effects.

OCCUPATIONAL EXPOSURE

Occupational exposure to toxic compounds is mainly chronic, continual exposure. The route of exposure is either via inhalation or skin contact. Consequently lung disease and dermatitis are common industrial diseases. Acute exposure may occur in the event of an accident such as an explosion, spillage or leakage or because of bad working practices. Cleaning out reactor vessels which have contained solvents may lead to acute toxicity due to excessive exposure for example.

ENVIRONMENTAL EXPOSURE

Effluents from factories, either gaseous or liquid may sometimes briefly, or more often continuously, contaminate our immediate environment and also more distant environments such as the seas and oceans or the atmosphere in other countries. This form of exposure is usually chronic but there have been isolated accidents at factories where acute exposure of humans outside the factory occurs such as at Bhopal and Seveso. Chronic exposure to gases such as sulphur dioxide, nitrogen oxides and carbon monoxide occurs in industrial areas and regions of heavy traffic and may cause acute irritation but the chronic toxic effects are largely unknown.

Environmental exposure is also important in relation to pesticides contaminating air, water and food. Large-scale spraying means that most people are exposed to pesticides or their residues both within their food and directly via the air.

ACCIDENTAL POISONING

This type of exposure is usually acute rather than chronic. Drugs, pesticides, household products and natural poisons may all be involved in this type of exposure, and children and the elderly are most commonly involved. Mistaken ingestion of a poisonous plant, cleaning fluid or drug falls into this category as does accidental ingestion of an excessive dose of a drug. Inhalation of fumes from fires and stoves is also an important cause of accidental poisoning.

INTENTIONAL POISONING

Fortunately homicide by poisoning is now relatively rare but suicide by poisoning is regrettably all too common. Drugs are commonly used but household products occasionally feature; both types are usually taken by mouth in these circumstances.

SELECTIVE TOXICITY

This is a very important concept in toxicology. It encompasses the differences in susceptibility to toxic effects between different species of animal or plant or between different cells, such as between tumour cells and normal cells.

It is in many cases a useful attribute which is utilized in the design of antibacterial drugs, pesticides or anti-cancer drugs. It is also of relevance to the prediction of toxicity in humans based on studies in another species.

The reasons for selective toxicity are various but can be divided into those due to differences in the absorption, distribution, metabolism and excretion of a chemical (toxicokinetics) or those due to biochemical differences affecting the presence of a receptor or target molecule (toxicodynamics).

For example the insect is more susceptible to the toxicity of **DDT** than mammalian organisms for two reasons. Firstly, the insect cuticle allows DDT to penetrate more readily than the mammalian skin. Secondly, the insect has a greater surface area to volume ratio and therefore absorbs relatively more DDT. Insects are more susceptible to some organophosphorus insecticides because the compound is metabolized by oxidative desulphuration to a compound that inhibits acetylcholinesterase, whereas in mammals enzymatic hydrolysis produces a metabolite that is more readily excreted but is not an inhibitor of acetylcholinesterase.

The rodenticide **norbormide** is active against rats because they possess a receptor in smooth muscle whereas humans, cats and dogs do not. Other **rodenticides** are based more simply on the fact that the rat does not have a vomit reflex, unlike many other mammals. Therefore after the oral ingestion of a poisonous chemical the rat is unable to rid itself of the substance by simply vomiting.

Penicillin is active against certain bacteria because it interferes with synthesis of the cell wall in multiplying bacteria but mammalian cells do not have a cell wall and therefore are not affected.

Dose–response relationship

'All substances are poisons; there is none which is not a poison. The right dose differentiates a poison and a remedy' **Paracelsus** (1493–1541).

Paracelsus was probably the first to recognize the concept that toxicity is a relative phenomenon and that it depends not only on the toxic properties but on the dose of the compound administered. This relationship between the dose of a compound and the response it elicits is a fundamental concept in toxicology. However, first we must consider the nature of the response itself. The toxic response that is simplest to observe is death but this is a crude parameter to measure. Another indicator of a toxic response is the presence of a pathological lesion such as liver cell necrosis. A more precisely measured response is a biochemical, pharmacological or chemical change.

We can distinguish between so-called '**all or none**' responses, such as death, and **graded** responses, such as the inhibition of an enzyme or the level of a marker of pathological damage. Both 'all or none' responses and graded responses can show a typical dose–response relation. In both cases there will be a dose at which there is no measurable effect and an upper dose where there is a maximal response. Very often in a toxicity study, either in whole animals or in isolated cells, lethality will be the first parameter of toxicity utilized but this gives little if any information about the underlying mechanism of toxicity. However, it is often important to know the limits of dosing in practical terms. Although it is not always necessary to know the lethal dose, it is important to know whether toxicity occurs at the dose or a multiple of the dose likely to be encountered by man or animals. However in certain situations it is extremely difficult or impossible to quantify the likely human dose and may be similarly difficult to extrapolate the likely effects in man from the available data (see also Chapter 12).

It should be noted that strictly speaking the word dose means the total amount of a substance administered to an organism whereas the term dosage includes a characteristic of the organism, typically body weight or surface area. Dosage is more precise, therefore, and can be related to other organisms, for example as mg substance/kg body weight. We can therefore talk about dosage–response relationships.

With 'all or none' responses (lethality for example) the normal way to determine and represent the dose–response relation is to determine the percentage of the animals or cells in a particular dosage or concentration group which show the response. This response is then plotted against the dosage or concentration

resulting in a typical sigmoid curve as illustrated in Figure 1.4. By using probit analysis the data can be plotted as a straight line.

When the response is a graded one the actual values measured are plotted against the dosage or concentration giving the same type of curve (Figure 1.4).

RECEPTORS

Although receptors are known to play an important part in pharmacological responses, with toxic effects at present the role of receptors seems more limited. There are, however, a few well understood receptor toxicant interactions such as that between the aryl hydrocarbon hydrolyase (Ah) receptor and a number of aromatic compounds such as dioxin (TCDD). It is possible that many toxic responses do not involve direct interactions with receptors in the pharmacological sense. It is more likely

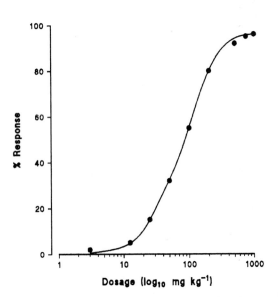

FIGURE 1.4 *A typical dose–response curve where the percentage response is plotted against the log of the dosage.*

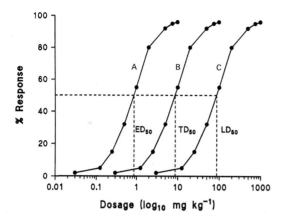

FIGURE 1.5 *Comparison of dose–response curves for efficacy (A), toxicity (B) and lethality (C). The effective, toxic or lethal dosage for 50% of the animals in the group can be estimated as shown. This graph shows the relationship between these parameters. The proximity of the ED_{50} and TD_{50} indicates the margin of safety of the compound.*

that toxic effects result from disturbances in enzyme function and metabolic pathways or damage to structures such as membranes and structural proteins. For some toxicants interaction with a particular protein or enzyme target does underlie the toxic effects. For example, the

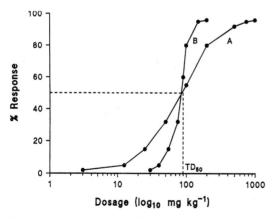

FIGURE 1.6 *Comparison of the toxicity of two compounds A and B. Although they both have the same TD_{50} compound A is more **potent** than compound B.*

toxicity of **cyanide** and **carbon monoxide** involve interaction with and disturbance of the function of important proteins (cytochrome aa_3 and haemoglobin, respectively, see Chapter 11). The toxic effects of these two compounds are a direct result of these interactions and the magnitude of the effects, it is assumed, depend on the number of molecules of toxicant bound to the protein. Thus, the more molecules of protein occupied by the chemical, the greater will be the toxic effect. There will be a concentration of the toxic compound at which all of the molecules of the receptor are occupied, however, and hence there will be no further increase in the toxic effect. This relationship gives rise to the classical dose–response curve (Figure 1.4). It is beyond the scope of this book to discuss this in more detail but several of the references in the bibliography may be consulted for more information.

Therefore the interpretation of the dose–response relationship is based on certain assumptions:

1   the response is proportional to the concentration at the target site;

2   the concentration at the target site is related to the dose;

3   the response is causally related to the compound administered.

The target site might be a receptor in which case the dose–response relationship may be similar to those observed with pharmacological effects. That is the receptor must be occupied by the toxic compound in order for there to be a response and there will be a point at which all the receptors are occupied, giving the maximum response.

However, with some toxic effects such as the liver necrosis caused by **paracetamol** or **carbon tetrachloride** for instance, although a dose-response relation can be demonstrated there may be no simple toxicant–receptor interaction which underlies the response.

Thus carbon tetrachloride is probably toxic as a result of a variety of effects including damage to membranes and inhibition of enzymes.

The later events or sequelae may indeed involve receptors which lead to genes being switched on or off or physiological events such as changes in blood pressure.

However, there are some well researched areas where receptors are crucially involved. One already alluded to are the biological effects of **dioxin** and related compounds. Here interaction with the Ah receptor directly leads to increased synthesis of cytochrome P450 (see below) and other effects. The toxicity of dioxin also seems to be related to the receptor interaction (see Chapter 9). The second well documented example of a receptor interaction is the peroxisome proliferators which interact with the **peroxisome proliferator activated receptor** (PPAR). (See Chapter 4.)

Although a toxic response may be observed after exposure to a substance at one particular dose, it is usual to demonstrate responses at several doses of the compound in question and that there is a relationship between the dose and the magnitude of the response.

The shape of the dose–response curve depends on the type of toxic effect measured

and the mechanism underlying it. For example, when **cyanide** reacts with cytochrome a_3 it binds irreversibly and curtails the function of the electron transport chain in the mitochondria. As this is a function vital to the life of the cell the dose–response curve for lethality is very steep for cyanide. The more precise the measurement made and the greater the number of determinations the more precise will be the curve and parameters derived from it.

Once a dose–response relationship has been demonstrated there are several parameters which can be derived from it. When lethality has been used as an endpoint, the LD_{50} can be determined (Figure 1.5). This is defined as the dosage of a substance which kills 50 per cent of the animals in a particular group, usually determined in an acute, single exposure study. It is not an exact value and in recent years there has been much discussion as to its usefulness and necessity in toxicology (see Chapter 12). The LD_{50} value may vary for the same compound between different groups of the same species of animal. The value itself is only of real use in a comparative sense, giving the toxicologist an idea of how toxic a compound is relative to other substances (Table 1.1, Figure 1.6) or enabling toxicity to be compared using various routes of administration (Table 1.2) or in different species for example (Table 1.3). It is also widely used for classification purposes,

TABLE 1.1 *Approximate LD_{50} values for a variety of chemical substances*

Compound	LD_{50} mg kg^{-1}
Ethanol	10,000
DDT	100
Nicotine	1
Tetrodotoxin	0.1
Dioxin	0.001
Botulinus toxin	0.00001

Source: T. A. Loomis (1974), *Essentials of Toxicology,* 2nd ed. (Philadelphia: Lea & Febiger).

TABLE 1.2 *Effect of route of administration on the toxicity of various compounds*

Route of administration	Pentobarbital[1] LD_{50} mg kg^{-1}	Isoniazid[1] LD_{50} mg kg^{-1}	Procaine[1] LD_{50} mg kg^{-1}	DFP[2] LD_{50} mg kg^{-1}
Oral	280	142	500	4.0
Subcutaneous	130	160	800	1.0
Intramuscular	124	140	630	0.9
Intraperitoneal	130	132	230	1.0
Intravenous	80	153	45	0.3

[1] Mouse toxicity data.
[2] Di-isopropylfluoro phosphate; Rabbit toxicity data.
Source: T. A. Loomis (1968), *Essentials of Toxicology* (Philadelphia: Lea & Febiger).

such as hazard warnings for example. Recently there has been a proposal by the British Toxicology Society for an alternative means of assessing the relative harmfulness of a compound which simply involves dosing a few animals with a range of doses and noting the responses. The chemical can then be classified as for example very toxic, toxic or not very toxic without the use of the LD_{50} test. (For a further discussion see Chapter 12.)

The ED_{50} (effective dosage for 50 per cent) and the TD_{50} (toxic dosage for 50 per cent) are similar parameters to the LD_{50} (Figure 1.5). They can be derived from the dose–response curve where the pharmacological effect or the toxic effect is plotted against dosage instead of lethality. The response can be either a quantal, all-or-none parameter such as death or the presence or absence of a tumour or a graded response such as the inhibition of an enzyme. So the response may be expressed as a proportion of the animals responding or the actual response, respectively.

TABLE 1.3 *Species differences in toxicity of ipomeanol*

	LD_{50} mg kg^{-1*}	Location of tissue damage		
		Liver	Kidney	Lung
Rabbit (New Zealand White)	40	−	−	+
Mouse (A/J Strain)	20	−	+	+
Rat (Fisher Strain)	12	−	−	+
Hamster (Syrian Golden)	140	+	−	+
Guinea Pig (Hartley)	30	−	−	+

*The ipomeanol was administered intraperitoneally in 25% aqueous propylene glycol to all species.
Source: J. S. Dutcher and M. R. Boyd (1979), *Biochem. Pharmacol.* **28**, 3367.

An important parameter in relation to drugs is the **Therapeutic Index**. This is determined from the ratio of either the LD_{50} or TD_{50} and the ED_{50}:

$$\frac{LD_{50}}{ED_{50}} \quad or \quad \frac{TD_{50}}{ED_{50}}$$

The larger the value the greater is the margin of safety between the dose of drug that is effective pharmacologically and the dose that is toxic. However, the therapeutic index does not give any indication of the shape of the dose–response curves and therefore possible overlap between the toxicity and therapeutic effect. Comparison of the dose–response curves will yield this information however (see Figure 1.5). Comparison of the dose–response curves for different compounds will indicate which is the more hazardous (see Figure 1.6).

SYNERGY AND POTENTIATION

In many cases exposure to chemicals occurs not to a single substance but to mixtures. This is especially so with drugs where a patient may be treated with several drugs at the same time. It may also be the case with exposure to environmental pollutants and industrial chemicals.

The effects of such mixtures may be different from the effects of each constituent separately and consequently may be unpredictable. The simplest situation is when each compound has similar effects and the overall toxicity of the mixture is the sum of the individual toxic effects. The effects are then described as additive. However, this may not necessarily be the case; for example, two substances may cause a greater response together than the sum of the individual responses. This is known as a **synergistic** effect. For example, **carbon tetrachloride** and **alcohol** together are more toxic to the liver than expected from the sum of the two indivi-

dual toxic effects. Potentiation is a similar effect except that the two compounds in question may have different toxic effects or only one may be toxic. For example, the drug **disulphiram** (antabuse) at non-toxic doses potentiates the toxicity of alcohol and is used for the treatment of alcohol abuse. The drug inhibits the enzyme aldehyde dehydrogenase and so allows an accumulation of acetaldehyde (ethanal) which has unpleasant effects.

The converse effect sometimes observed is a decreased response from a mixture compared with the constituents. This is referred to as antagonism. After repeated exposure, the response may lessen despite similar dosage; tolerance has developed. This may be due to induction of enzymes (see Chapter 2) and hence increased metabolism or to a change in the response or number of receptors. Alternatively repeated exposure can result in accumulation and an exaggerated response.

Such effects must of course be considered when assessing risk from exposure to chemicals and attempting to predict effects.

THE THRESHOLD DOSE AND NO OBSERVED ADVERSE EFFECT LEVEL (NOAEL)

For some compounds and types of toxic effect there will clearly be a dose below which no effect or response is measurable. There is thus a threshold dose. This can be clearly demonstrated for quantal responses such as lethality, the presence or absence of a pathological lesion or a teratogenic effect for example. This means that there will be a dose at which the response does not occur in any individuals in the population (Figure 1.7). Alternatively the concept could apply to a variable response such as enzyme inhibition which can be measured with increasing concentrations of the compound in question.

The concept of a threshold dose for the toxic effect is an important one in toxicology because it implies that there is a 'no observed adverse effect level', or NOAEL. While this is generally accepted for most types of toxic effect, for chemical carcinogenesis mediated via a genotoxic mechanism this is a controversial issue. In the case of such carcinogens the dose–response curve when extrapolated seems to cross the x-axis at the origin rather than at some positive value or dosage level (Figure 1.7). This means that there is a response at all exposure levels tested and so within the limits of the analytical techniques available no safe exposure level can be set with confidence (see Chapter 12).

The NOAEL is important for setting exposure limits. For example, the **acceptable daily intake (ADI)** is based on the NOAEL. This is a factor used to determine the safe intake for food additives and contaminants such as pesticides and residues of veterinary drugs and, hence, to establish the safe level in food (see Chapter 12).

In the industrial setting, exposure is regulated in a similar way and the term used is the **Threshold Limit Value (TLV; USA)** or **Maximum Exposure Limit (MEL; UK)** which is usually based on exposure for an eight-hour working day (see also Chapters 6 and 12). The NOAEL is usually based on animal toxicity studies with the compound in question, using the most sensitive species and most discriminating test.

It is clear therefore that the dose–response relationship is a crucial concept in toxicology.

Summary and learning objectives

In this chapter you will have learnt about the *origins* of toxicology in antiquity, mainly in relation to intentional poisoning. Some notable figures were mentioned especially Maimonides, Paracelsus, Orfila and Bernard. These individuals all helped toxicology develop from an art into a science. The breadth and scope of toxicology is illustrated by the variety of *types of toxic substance* to which we are exposed, ranging from drugs, food additives, industrial chemicals, environmental pollutants, household poisons to natural toxins.

This is also underlined by the *types of exposure* such as occupational, accidental or intentional. Toxicity may be *selective*, affecting different cell types (tumour vs. normal) or species (mammals vs. microorganisms) differently. This concept is used for the design of anticancer drugs, antibiotics and pesticides.

One of the most important concepts for you to remember because it underlies toxicology, is the *dose–response relationship*. It was first formulated by Paracelsus in his famous phrase 'All substances are poisons, there is none that is not;

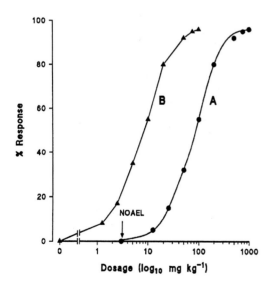

FIGURE 1.7 *Comparison of the dose–response relationships for two compounds A and B. For compound B there is a response at any dose with no threshold. For compound A there is a dose or threshold level below which there is a No Observed Adverse Effect (NOAEL). For compounds such as B there is no safe dose.*

the right dose distinguishes a poison from a remedy.' This relationship between the dose of the toxicant and the effect it produces or the toxic response is based on three premises: that the response is proportional to concentration of toxicant at the target site; that the concentration of toxicant is proportional to the dose; that the response is causally related to the toxicant. The target site may be a *receptor* with a specific function (e.g. Ah receptor) or an enzyme (e.g. cytochrome aa_3) or a protein (e.g. haemoglobin). However, receptors are not always involved in toxic reactions.

Exposure to chemicals may be to mixtures when *synergy* or *potentiation* may occur.

Several important parameters can be calculated from the dose–response curve. These are the No Observed Adverse Effect Level (*NOAEL*), which is determined from the bottom of the curve, the maximal effect, and the dose causing a 50 per cent effect or which affects 50 per cent of the animals dosed. This could be a biochemical or pharmacological effect (ED_{50}) a toxic effect (TD_{50}) or a lethal effect (LD_{50}). From these can be determined the *therapeutic index* (TD_{50}/ED_{50}) and the margin of safety (TD_1/ED_{99}).

From the NOAEL can be determined the Acceptable Daily Intake (ADI) or Tolerable Daily Intake (TDI) that is involved in the risk assessment of food additives or food contaminants, respectively.

Questions

Q1.   Choose one answer which you think is the most appropriate.
A particular dose of a chemical A, is toxic to animals *in vivo*. Another chemical, B, is not toxic even when given at doses several orders of magnitude higher than the dose of A. When A and B are given together at the same dose, the toxic response is greater than that of the dose of A alone.
Is this an example of:

a   antagonism
b   synergism
c   additivity
d   potentiation
e   none of the above.

Q2.   Which information may be gained from an acute toxicity study?

a   the No Effect Level
b   the LD_{50}
c   the therapeutic index
d   the target organ
e   all of the above.

Q3.   The therapeutic index is usually defined as?

a TD_{50}/LD_{50}
b ED_{50}/LD_{50}
c LD_{50}/ED_{50}
d ED_{50}/TD_{50}
e LD_1/ED_{99}.

SHORT ANSWER QUESTIONS

Q4.   Explain the following:

a TD_{50}
b   dose–response relationship
c   therapeutic index
d   NOAEL.

Q5.   Explain selective toxicity using examples.

Q6.   Write notes on the following:

a ED_{50}
b   ADI
c   margin of safety

Bibliography

ALBERT, A. (1979) *Selective Toxicity,* London: Chapman & Hall. Somewhat idiosyncratic but nevertheless useful text.

ALBERT, A. (1987) *Xenobiosis,* London: Chapman & Hall. Similar to *Selective Toxicity.*

ANDERSON, D. and CONNING, D. M. (Eds) (1993) *Experimental Toxicology. The Basic Issues,* Cambridge: Royal Society of Chemistry.

BALLANTYNE, B., MARRS, T. and SYVERSEN, T. L. M. (1999) Fundamentals of Toxicology, in *General and Applied Toxicology*, Ballantyne, B., Marrs, T. and Syversen, T. L. M. (Eds) 2nd edition, Macmillan: Basingstoke. The book is a comprehensive reference text.

BORZELLECA, J. F. (2001) The Art, the Science and the Seduction of Toxicology: An Evolutionary Development, in *Principles and Methods of Toxicology*, A. W. Hayes (Ed.), 4th edition, Philadelphia: Taylor & Francis. Another comprehensive reference text.

CARSON, R. (1965) *Silent Spring,* London: Chapman & Hall.

DEICHMANN, W. B., HENSCHLER, D., HOLMSTEDT, B. and KEIL, G. (1986) What is there that is not a poison: a study of the Third Defense by Paracelsus, *Archives of Toxicology,* **58**, 207.

EATON, D. L. and KLAASSEN, C. D. (1996) Principles of Toxicology, in *Casarett and Doull's Toxicology, The Basic Science of Poisons,* C. D. Klaassen (Ed.), 5th edition, New York: McGraw-Hill.

EFRON, E. (1984) *The Apocalyptics, Cancer and the Big Lie,* New York: Simon & Shuster.

GALLO, M. A. (1996) History and Scope of Toxicology, in *Casarett and Doull's Toxicology, The Basic Science of Poisons,* C. D. Klaassen (Ed.), 5th edition, New York: McGraw-Hill. This book is also a comprehensive reference text.

HODGSON, E. and LEVI, P. E. (1987) *A Textbook of Modern Toxicology,* Barking: Elsevier.

KOEMAN, J. H. (1996) Toxicology: History and Scope of the Field, in *Toxicology: Principles and Practice*, R. J. M. Niesink, J. de Vries and M. A. Hollinger (Eds), CRC Press and Open University of the Netherlands. Comprehensive but also includes some useful examples and questions and answers.

LOOMIS, T. A. and HAYES, A. W. (1996) *Loomis's Essentials of Toxicology*, 4th edition, San Diego: Academic Press.

LU, F. C. (1996) *Basic Toxicology*, 3rd edition, New York: Taylor & Francis. Comprehensive but concise coverage of the subject.

MANN, J. (1994) *Murder, Magic and Medicine,* Oxford: Oxford University Press.

MCCLELLAN, R. O. (Ed.) (1971) *Critical Reviews in Toxicology*, Boca Raton, Florida: CRC Press. A series of in depth review articles.

MORIARTY, F. (1999) *Ecotoxicology: The Study of Pollutants in Ecosystems*, 3rd edition, London: Academic Press.

MUNTER, S. (Ed.) (1966) *Treatise on Poisons and Their Antidotes*, vol. II of the Medical Writings of Moses Maimonides, Philadelphia: J. P. Lippincott.

PRATT, W. B. and TAYLER, P. (Eds). (1990) *Principles of Drug Action: The Basis of Pharmacology*, 3rd edition, New York: Churchill Livingstone. The pharmacology and kinetics sections are useful with some coverage of toxicology.

SHAW, I. C. and CHADWICK, J. (1998) *Principles of Environmental Toxicology*, London: Taylor & Francis.

STACEY, N. H. (Ed.) (1993) *Occupational Toxicology*, London: Taylor & Francis.

THOMPSON, C. J. S. (1931) *Poisons and Poisoners,* London: H. Shaylor.

WALKER, C. H., HOPKIN, S. P., SIBLY, R. M. and PEAKALL, D. B. (2001) *Principles of Ecotoxicology*, 2nd edition, London: Taylor & Francis. An excellent text on this aspect of toxicology.

WEXLER, P. (1987) *Information Sources in Toxicology*, 2nd edition, New York: Elsevier.

WORLD HEALTH ORGANISATION (1978) *Principles and Methods for Evaluating the Toxicity of Chemicals. Part I. Environmental Health Criteria 6,* Geneva: WHO.

ZBINDEN, G. (1988) Biopharmaceutical studies, a key to better toxicology, *Xenobiotica,* **18**, suppl. 1, 9.

CHAPTER — 2

Disposition of toxic compounds

Chapter outline

In this chapter the disposition of chemicals in biological systems will be discussed:

- The absorption of toxic compounds into biological systems

  - the cell membrane

  - transport of toxicants through cell membranes

  - sites of absorption of toxic substances and factors affecting absorption

    skin

    lungs

    gastrointestinal tract

- The distribution of toxic compounds in the body

  - volume of distribution

  - plasma level

  - half life

  - area under the curve

  - plasma protein binding

  - site of action

  - accumulation

- The excretion of toxic compounds and factors affecting excretion

  - urinary excretion

  - biliary excretion

  - excretion via lungs

The disposition of a toxic compound in a biological system may be divided into four phases: absorption, distribution, metabolism and excretion. These four phases are interrelated:

Absorption → Distribution → Metabolism
                    ↘   ↗
                     Excretion

and we shall consider each of them in turn.

1   size

2   lipid solubility

3   similarity to endogenous molecules

4   polarity/charge

Absorption of toxic compounds

Before a substance can exert a toxic effect it must come into contact with a biological system. Indeed the means, the rate and the site of absorption may all be important factors in the eventual toxicity of a compound. There are several sites for first contact between a toxic compound and a biological system but absorption necessarily involves the passage across cell membranes whichever site is involved. Consequently it is important to consider first the structure and characteristics of biological membranes in order to understand the passage of substances across them.

Membranes are composed mainly of **phospholipids** and **proteins** with the lipids arranged as a **bilayer** interspersed with proteins as shown in Figure 2.1. The particular proteins and phospholipids incorporated into the membrane vary depending on the cell type in which the membrane is located. The proteins may be structural or have a specific function, such as a carrier for membrane transport. The phospholipids may have one of several polar head groups (Figure 2.2) and the fatty acid chains may be saturated, unsaturated or a mixture of both. The degree of saturation will influence the fluidity of the membrane. Cholesterol esters and certain carbohydrates are also found in some membranes.

The structure of biological membranes determines their function and characteristics. The most important feature from a toxicological point of view is that they are selectively permeable. Only certain substances are able to pass through them, depending on particular physicochemical characteristics:

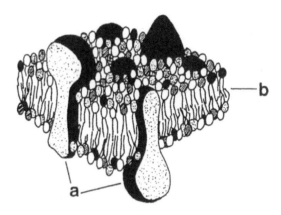

FIGURE 2.1   *The three-dimensional structure of the animal cell membrane. Proteins (a) are interspersed in the phospholipid bilayer (b).*

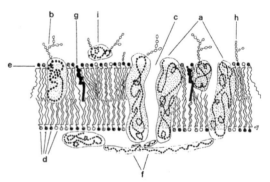

FIGURE 2.2   *The molecular arrangement of the cell membrane. a: integral proteins; b: glycoprotein; c: pore formed from integral protein; d: various phospholipids with saturated fatty acid chains; e: phospholipid with unsaturated fatty acid chains; f: network proteins; g: cholesterol; h: glycolipid; i: peripheral protein. There are four different phospholipids: phosphatidyl serine; phosphatidyl choline; phosphatidyl ethanolamine; sphingomyelin represented as* ○; ◌; ◪; ●. *The stippled area of the protein represents the hydrophobic portion.*

The lipid solubility of a chemical substance is usually represented by its **partition coefficient**: the oil/water partition coefficient is the comparative solubility of the chemical in aqueous versus organic solvents. It can be simply determined by shaking a solution of the chemical in water or buffer with an organic solvent such as chloroform or a biologically more relevant liquid such as olive oil. The concentration remaining in the aqueous phase and that in the organic phase are then measured and compared. The greater the lipid solubility of a compound, the greater is the value.

The ways in which foreign substances may pass through biological membranes are as follows:

1 **filtration through pores**

2 **passive diffusion through the membrane phospholipid**

3 **active transport**

4 **facilitated diffusion**

5 **phago/pinocytosis**

1 *Filtration.* Small molecules may pass through **pores** in the membrane formed by proteins. This movement will occur down a concentration gradient and may include substances such as ethanol and urea.

2 *Passive diffusion.* This is probably the most important mechanism of absorption for foreign and toxic compounds. For passive diffusion to occur certain conditions are required:

   a there must be a **concentration gradient** across the membrane
   b the foreign molecule must be **lipid soluble**
   c the compound must be **non-ionized**

These principles are embodied in the **pH-partition theory**: only non-ionized lipid soluble compounds will be absorbed by passive diffusion down a concentration gradient. Furthermore certain factors affect the rate at which foreign compounds passively diffuse. This rate of diffusion is described by **Ficks Law**:

$$\text{Rate of diffusion} = KA(C_2 - C_1)$$

where A is the surface area, C_2 is the concentration outside and C_1 the concentration inside the membrane, and K is a constant.

The above relationship applies to a system at constant temperature and for diffusion over unit distance. The concentration gradient is represented by $(C_2 - C_1)$. Passive diffusion is a **first order process**, that is the rate of diffusion is *proportional* to the concentration.

Normally biological systems are dynamic and the concentration on the inside of the membrane is continually reducing as the foreign compound is being removed by blood flow and possibly ionization (Figure 2.3). Consequently there is always a concentration gradient towards the inside of the membrane. As well as a concentration gradient, lipid solubility and ionization and, hence, the pH of the particular tissue fluid are also factors in passive diffusion. Lipid soluble compounds are able to pass across biological membranes by dissolution in the phospholipid and movement down the concentration gradient. Ionizable compounds will only do this if they are in the non-ionized form. The degree of ionization can be calculated from the **Henderson Hasselbach** equation:

$$pH = pK_a + \frac{\text{Log}[A^-]}{[HA]}$$

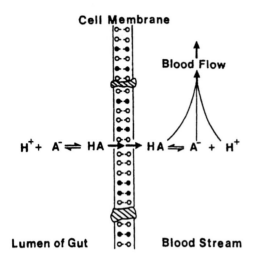

Cell Membrane

Blood Flow

$$H^+ + A^- \rightleftharpoons HA \rightarrow HA \rightleftharpoons A^- + H^+$$

Lumen of Gut   **Blood Stream**

FIGURE 2.3 *Role of blood flow and ionization in the absorption of foreign compounds. Both blood flow and ionization create a gradient across the membrane.*

where pK_a is the dissociation constant for the acid, HA. The ionization of an acid and base are shown in Figure 2.4. The role of ionization will be discussed more fully when the gastrointestinal tract is considered.

3   *Active transport.* Active transport of compounds across membranes has several important features:

a   a specific membrane **carrier** is required
b   metabolic **energy** is necessary to operate the system
c   the process may be **inhibited** by metabolic poisons
d   the process may be **saturated** at high substrate concentrations and hence is **zero order** rather than first order
e   transport occurs against a **concentration gradient**
f   similar substrates may **compete** for uptake

There are various kinds of active transport systems which involve carrier molecules operating in different ways. These are **uniports**, **symports** and **antiports**. The uniport transports one molecule in a single direction. Symports and antiports transport two molecules in the same or opposite directions respectively.

This type of membrane transport is normally specific for endogenous and nutrient substances but analogues and similar molecules or ions may be transported by the system. For example, the drug **fluorouracil**, an analogue of uracil and **lead** ions are absorbed from the gut by specific transport systems.

4   *Facilitated diffusion.* This has the following salient features:

a   a specific membrane **carrier** is required
b   a **concentration gradient** across the membrane is necessary
c   the process may be **saturated** by high substrate concentrations

Unlike active transport, no energy expenditure is necessary. This type of transport system also normally applies to endogenous substances and normal nutrients but may apply to foreign compounds which are structurally similar to an endogenous compound. The transport of glucose from the cells of the intestine into the bloodstream involves this type of system.

5   *Phagocytosis and pinocytosis.* These involve the **invagination** of the membrane to enclose a particle or droplet respectively. This is the mechanism by which particles of insoluble substances such as **uranium dioxide and asbestos** are absorbed into the lungs.

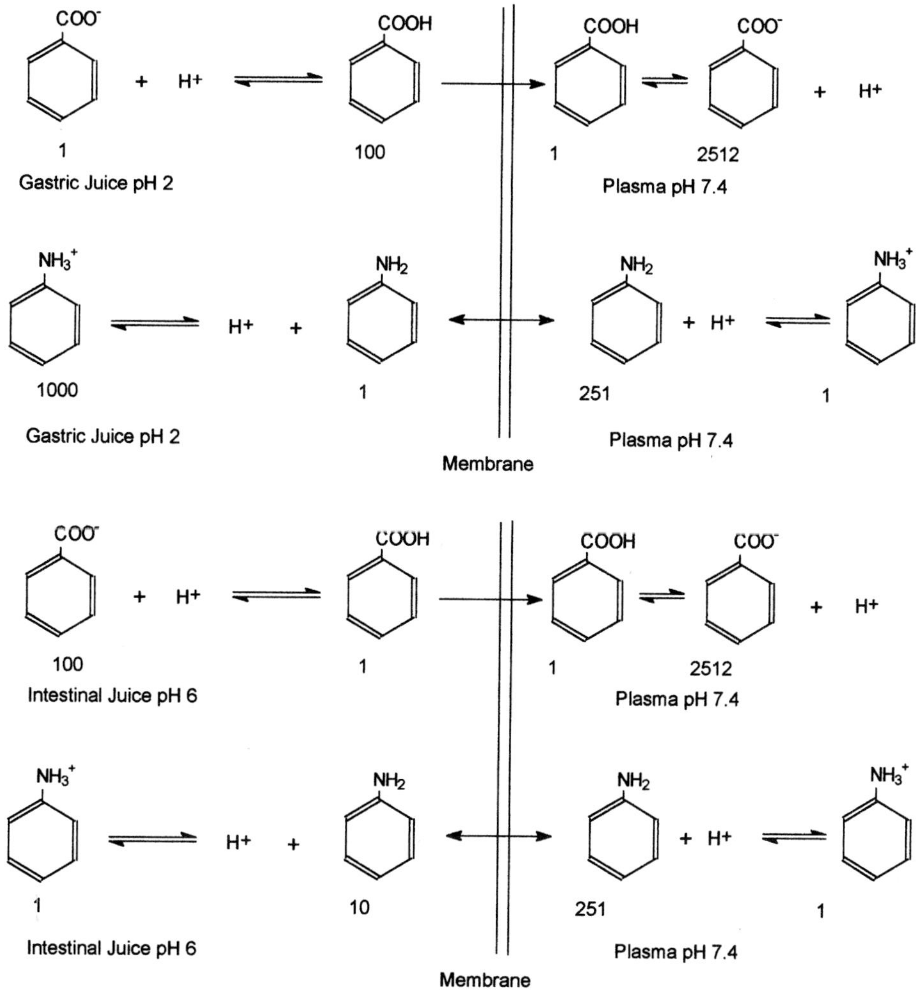

FIGURE 2.4 *Ionization of an acid and base in the stomach and intestine.*
From Timbrell, J. A., Principles of Biochemical Toxicology, *Taylor & Francis, London, 2000.*

SITES OF ABSORPTION

There are three major sites for the absorption of foreign compounds: the skin, lungs and gastro-intestinal tract. The gastrointestinal tract is the most important in toxicology as most foreign compounds are ingested orally. The lungs are clearly important for all airborne compounds whereas the skin is only rarely a significant site for absorption.

Skin

The skin is constantly exposed to foreign compounds such as gases, solvents, and substances in solution, and so absorption through the skin is potentially an important route. However, although the skin has a large **surface area** for absorption, its structure is such as to present a barrier to absorption. This is because there is an outer layer of dead cells, a poor blood supply, and the outer cells of the epidermis are packed with **keratin** (Figure 2.5). Although the dermis below is vascularized, it is several cells thick and this will also inhibit absorption.

Absorption through the skin is mainly limited to lipid soluble compounds such as solvents. Fatalities have occurred, however, following absorption of toxic compounds by this route, such as with the insecticide **parathion**.

Lungs

Exposure to toxic compounds via the lungs is toxicologically more important than via the skin. The air we breathe may contain many foreign substances. These may be gases (**carbon monoxide**), vapours from solvents (**methylene chloride**), aerosols or particulate matter (**asbestos**) in an industrial or other workplace environment. Also, the air in an urban or home environment may contain noxious gases (**sul-**

phur dioxide and **nitrogen oxides**), particulates (**fibre glass** and **pollen**), and possibly solvent vapours and aerosols from home use. The lungs have a very large **surface area**, around 50–100 m² in man, they have an excellent blood supply, and the barrier between the air in the alveolus and the blood stream may be as little as two cell membranes thick (Figure 2.6). Consequently absorption from the lungs is rapid and efficient. Two factors which affect absorption via the lungs are blood flow and breathing rate. For compounds with low solubility in blood the absorption will be mainly dependent on the rate of blood flow. For compounds with high solubility in blood the absorption will be mainly dependent on the breathing rate. The rapid rate of blood flow means that foreign substances are continually removed from the absorption site and, therefore, there is always a concentration gradient.

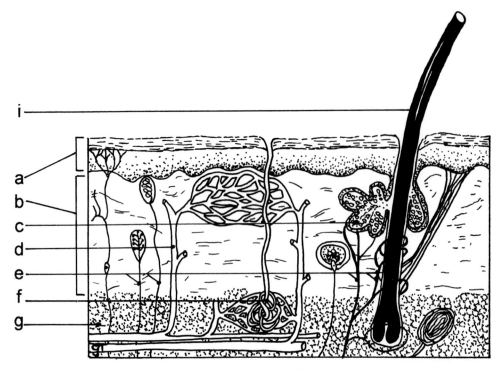

FIGURE 2.5 *The structure of mammalian skin. a: epidermis; b: dermis; c: sebaceous gland; d: capillary; e: nerve fibre; f: sweat gland; g: adipose tissue; i: hair. Drawing by C. J. Waterfield.*

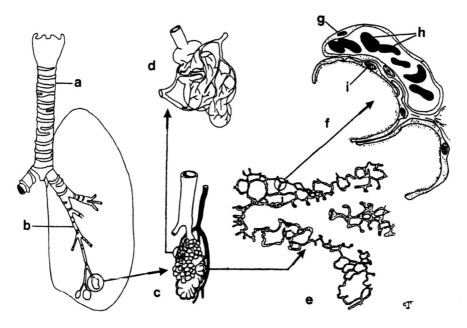

FIGURE 2.6 *The structure of the mammalian respiratory system. a: trachea; b: bronchiole; c: alveolar sac with blood supply; d: arrangement of blood vessels around alveoli; e: arrangement of cells and airspaces in alveoli showing the large surface area available for absorption; f: cellular structure of alveolus showing the close association between the endothelial cell of the capillary, g, with erythrocytes, h, and the epithelial cell of the alveolar sac, i. The luminal side of the epithelial cell is bathed in fluid which also facilitates absorption and gaseous exchange.*

Reaction with plasma proteins and for gases particularly dissolution in the plasma may also be factors.

Small, lipid soluble compounds, such as solvents, will be readily absorbed from the alveolus. For compounds which are absorbed via the lungs it is a very efficient and rapid route of entry to the body. Compounds in solution and particles may be absorbed by pinocytosis and phagocytosis respectively. For example, **uranium dioxide** particles, which are insoluble, are absorbed via the lungs and cause kidney damage. **Lead** is also absorbed in the particulate form from the air via the lungs. The size of particle is a major factor in determining where in the respiratory system it is deposited and whether it is absorbed. For example, lead particles of 0.25 μm diameter are absorbed but uranium dioxide particles of more than 3 μm diameter are not.

Gastrointestinal tract

Numerous foreign substances are taken in via the diet, while many drugs are normally taken by mouth, and various poisonous substances taken either accidentally or intentionally are usually ingested **orally**. Consequently the gastrointestinal tract is a very important site of absorption for foreign compounds.

The internal environment of the gastrointestinal tract varies throughout its length, particularly with regard to the **pH**. Substances taken orally first come into contact with the lining of the mouth (buccal cavity), where the pH is normally around 7 in man, but more alkaline in some other species such as the rat. The next region of importance is the stomach where the pH is around 2 in man and certain other mammals. The substance may remain in the stomach for some time particularly if it is taken in with food. In the small intestine where the pH is around 6, there is a good blood supply and a large surface area due to folding of the lining and the presence of villi (Figure 2.7).

Due to the change in pH in the gastrointestinal tract different substances may be absorbed in different areas depending on their **physico-chemical characteristics**. Lipid soluble, non-ionized compounds will be absorbed along the whole length of the tract, but ionizable substances generally will only be absorbed by **passive diffusion** if they are **non-ionized** at the pH of the particular site and are also **lipid soluble**. The Henderson Hasselbach equation can be used to calculate the extent of ionization of aniline (a weak base) and benzoic acid (a weak acid) at the particular pH prevailing in the stomach and small intestine. It can be seen (Figure 2.4) that **weak acids** should be absorbed in the **stomach** and **weak bases** in the **small intestine**.

However in practice weak acids are also absorbed in the small intestine due to the influence of blood flow and plasma pH. Although they exist mainly in the ionized form in the small intestine (Figure 2.4), the non-ionized form passing into the blood will immediately be removed by:

1 **blood flow**, and

2 **ionization** at pH 7.4.

These two factors ensure that weak acids are absorbed to a certain extent in the small intestine if they have not been fully absorbed in the stomach.

Another factor which may affect absorption from the gastrointestinal tract is the presence of **food**. This may facilitate absorption if the substance in question dissolves in any fat present in

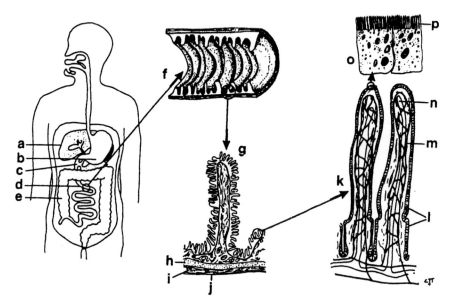

FIGURE 2.7 *The mammalian gastrointestinal tract showing important features of the small intestine, the major site of absorption for orally administered compounds. a: liver; b: stomach; c: duodenum; d: ileum; e: colon; f: longitudinal section of the ileum showing folding which increases surface area; g: detail of fold showing villi with circular and longitudinal muscles, h and i respectively, bounded by the serosal membrane, j; k: detail of villi showing network of capillaries, m, lacteals, n, and epithelial cells, l; o: detail of epithelial cells showing brush border or microvilli, p. The folding, vascularization and microvilli all facilitate absorption of substances from the lumen.*

the foodstuff but may delay absorption if the compound is only absorbed in the small intestine, as food **prolongs gastric emptying** time.

When drugs and other foreign compounds are administered the vehicle used to suspend or dissolve the compound may have a major effect on the eventual toxicity by affecting the rate of absorption and distribution.

The site of absorption itself may be important in the eventual toxicity because of the blood supply to that site as discussed in the next section.

The site of absorption and exposure to compounds may also be important in the fate of the compound. For example, the acidic conditions of the stomach may cause the substance to **hydrolyze**, or poisons such as **snake venom** may be **inactivated**. The **bacteria** in the gastrointestinal tract may metabolize foreign compounds as may enzymes in the gut wall. In the lungs phagocytosis sequesters some inert substances, such as particles of **asbestos** which can remain in the lung tissue for long periods of time with eventual toxic consequences.

Distribution of toxic compounds

After a foreign compound has been absorbed it passes into the **bloodstream**. The part of the vascular system into which the compound is absorbed will depend on the site of absorption. Absorption through the skin leads to the **peripheral blood** supply, whereas the major **pulmonary circulation** will be involved if the compound is airborne and hence absorbed through the lungs. For the majority of compounds **oral** absorption will be followed by entry of the compound into the **portal vein** supplying the liver with blood from the gastrointestinal tract.

Once in the bloodstream the compound will then be distributed around the body and be diluted by the blood. Depending on the **physico-chemical properties** of the compound it may then be distributed into the tissues. As with the absorption of foreign compounds, distribution into particular tissues involves crossing biological **membranes** and the principles which have already been discussed earlier in the chapter again apply. Only the **non-ionized** form of compounds will pass out of the bloodstream into tissues by passive diffusion. Specific transport systems may operate for certain compounds, and phagocytosis and pinocytosis may transport large molecules, particles or solutions of large molecules. The **concentration** of the compound in the plasma and the plasma level profile (Figure 2.8) will reflect the distribution. For example, compounds which are distributed into all tissues, such as lipid soluble solvents like carbon tetrachloride, will tend to have low plasma concentrations, whereas substances which are ionized at the pH of the plasma and which do not readily distribute into tissues, may have much higher plasma concentrations. This can be quantified as the parameter known as apparent **volume of distribution**, V_D:

$$V_D(L) = \frac{\text{Dose} \qquad (mg)}{\text{Plasma concentration}\,(mg\ L^{-1})}$$

(There are other means of determining V_D which the interested reader may find in more advanced texts.)

This is the volume of body fluids into which the particular substance is apparently distributed. The determination is analogous to dissolving a known amount (dose) of a substance in an unknown volume of water (body fluids). A knowledge of the concentration of compound in the water (plasma level) allows us to determine the volume of water.

The volume of distribution may sometimes indicate that a foreign compound is localized in a particular tissue or is confined mainly to the plasma. Thus, if a substance distributes mainly into **adipose tissue**, the plasma concentration will be very low and from the above formula it can be seen that the volume of distribution will be large. The substance is not necessarily evenly distributed in body water however and may reach high concentrations in one particular tissue or organ.

The concentration of a chemical in the blood plasma and its change over time (Figure 2.8) is a reflection of the absorption, distribution, metabolism and excretion of the chemical. For example, after a drug is taken orally, the **plasma level** profile will be different from the profile of a drug given intravenously (Figure 2.9). The plasma level of a chemical and its change over time are vitally important pieces of information for a toxicologist. This is because:

a   it reflects the concentration of the chemical in the tissues more readily than does the dose of the chemical which may be incompletely absorbed;

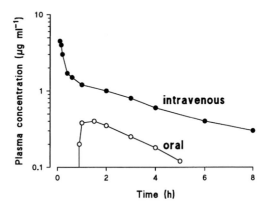

FIGURE 2.9 *The plasma level profile of a foreign compound after oral and intravenous administration. The marked difference in the areas under the curves (AUC) may indicate that first pass metabolism is occurring.*

b   it may reflect the concentration of the chemical at the target site;

c   it is necessary in order to calculate parameters such as **half-life**, V_D, **AUC** and **body burden**;

d   it may indicate the type of distribution which the compound is undergoing (i.e. which compartments it is distributed to);

e   the plasma level when plotted against time gives an indication of the duration of significant exposure (area under the curve or AUC; see Figure 2.8).

An indication of the overall exposure of the animal is given by the body burden, determined by V_D × plasma concentration.

For a drug, the plasma level indicates whether it has reached the therapeutic concentration and if so how quickly and for how long or whether the drug has reached a toxic concentration (see Figure 2.8).

The **half-life** ($t_{\frac{1}{2}}$) of the chemical in the blood can be calculated from the graph of the plasma

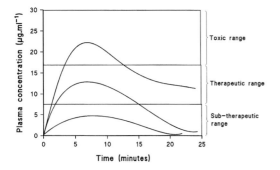

FIGURE 2.8 *The blood or plasma level profiles of three different doses of a drug after oral ingestion by an animal. The doses given are sub-therapeutic, therapeutic and toxic. The plasma level is plotted on a linear scale. The area under each curve (AUC) represents the overall exposure of the animal.*

level plotted against time (if the plasma level is plotted on a log scale) (see Figure 2.9). The half-life is defined as the time taken for the plasma concentration to decrease by half and is determined by metabolism and excretion. Clearly, a substance with a long half-life will be in contact with the biological system for longer than a compound with a short half-life and is an indication of the likelihood of a substance accumulating with repeated or chronic dosing. It is normally a constant value but if not, one or both of the processes that determine the decline in plasma level, metabolism or excretion, is saturable.

The plasma level of a chemical is important information for the treatment of patients suffering overdoses of drugs. Thus it allows the clinical toxicologist to know the exact exposure rather than have to estimate an overdose and to estimate the elimination rate and time of dosing. It is important information for an experimental toxicologist who needs to know that absorption of the chemical has occurred and to what extent the organs and tissues of the animal have been exposed. It also allows the half-life to be calculated, which lets the experimental toxicologist design repeated dose studies.

It will be clear from Figure 2.9 that the **AUC** after oral dosing is much less than that after intravenous dosing. This may be because the drug or other compound is metabolized during the absorption process either in the gastrointestinal tract or in the liver. This is known as '**first-pass metabolism**' and means that less of the parent compound reaches the circulation after oral dosing.

Another indicator of the ability of the body to eliminate the compound is the total body clearance which is calculated as shown:

$$\frac{\text{dose}}{\text{AUC}}$$

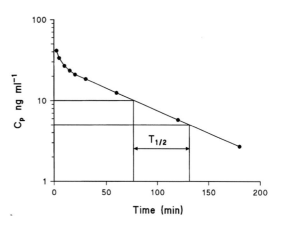

FIGURE 2.10 *Plasma level of a chemical after intravenous administration. The plasma level is plotted on a log scale. The half life ($T_\frac{1}{2}$) can be determined as shown. The elimination rate constant (k_{el}) can be determined from the slope of the linear part of the line.*

(The units are ml min^{-1} if the dose is in mg and the plasma concentration is plotted as mg ml^{-1} against minutes.)

Another aspect of the distribution phase which may have important toxicological implications is the interaction of foreign compounds with **proteins** in plasma and various macromolecules in other tissues. Many foreign compounds bind to plasma proteins non-covalently and in doing so their distribution is altered. Distribution from the blood into the tissues is reduced by binding to such proteins as the foreign compound is now attached to a large molecule which limits its passage across membranes unless a specific transport system exists. Binding can also limit excretion as will be discussed later. Foreign compounds in plasma often exist in equilibrium between the bound and unbound form and the extent of binding and the tightness of that binding varies between different compounds. Binding may involve **ionic** forces, **hydrogen bonding, hydrophobic bonding** and **Van der Waals** forces. Foreign compounds bind most commonly to **albumin** but some, such as **DDT**, which are lipophilic may associate extensively with plasma **lipoproteins**.

Distribution of foreign compounds to those tissues which may be the site of action is a particularly important aspect of their toxicology. For example, **barbiturates** act on the central nervous system and so must enter the brain in order to have a pharmacological, and if exaggerated, toxic, effect. The entry of substances into the brain is less readily attainable than passage into other tissues because of the so-called **blood-brain barrier**. This is due to the nature of the capillaries serving the brain. These are surrounded by cells which do not allow the ready passage of substances into the central nervous system. Lipid soluble compounds such as some of the barbiturates will enter the brain by passive diffusion. However, some barbiturates, such as phenobarbital, are weak acids and so ionize. In the treatment of barbiturate **poisoning** this ionization is utilized by increasing the plasma pH with infusions of **sodium bicarbonate**. This increases the ionization of the barbiturate in the plasma, changes the equilibrium and so causes more unionized drug to diffuse out of the tissues, including the brain, into the plasma. Another compound which is known to be toxic due to its effect on the central nervous system is **methyl mercury**, a lipophilic mercury derivative which is able to cross the blood-brain barrier.

Lipophilic foreign compounds localize particularly in body fat, sometimes to the extent that the plasma level is hardly detectable and the V_D is very large. For example, **polybrominated biphenyls**, substances once used extensively in industry, are very persistent and highly fat soluble. This localization in body fat resulting in very long whole body half-lives may have important toxicological consequences. The drug **thiopental**, a barbiturate anaesthetic which is very lipid soluble, has an extremely

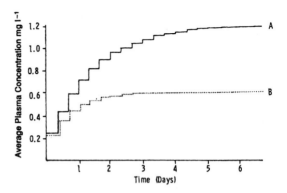

FIGURE 2.11 *Accumulation of two compounds after multiple dosing. Compound A has a half-life of 24 hours, compound B of 12 hours. Dosing interval is 8 hours.*
From Timbrell, J. A., Principles of Biochemical Toxicology, *Taylor & Francis, London, 2000.*

rapid onset of action due to its ability to enter the brain very quickly.

Some toxic foreign compounds are chronically ingested or there is continuous exposure to them over shorter periods and this may alter their disposition. If the dosing interval is shorter than the **half-life** the compound will accumulate in the animal (Figure 2.11). The blood and tissue level may increase disproportionately and dramatically under certain circumstances, such as where excretion or metabolism is saturated. Otherwise the plateau level reached in the plasma is proportional to the plasma half-life, so that compounds with long half-lives could accumulate to significant levels on repeated dosing or exposure despite the low level of each dose or exposure (Figure 2.11).

Excretion of toxic compounds

The elimination of toxic substances from the body is clearly an important determinant of their biological effect; rapid elimination will reduce the likelihood of toxicity occurring and reduce the duration of the biological effect. In the case of a toxic effect, removal of the compound may help to reduce the extent of damage.

The elimination of foreign compounds is reflected in either the plasma half-life or the whole body half-life. However, the plasma half-life also reflects metabolism and distribution as well as excretion. The **whole body half-life** is the time required for half of the compound to be eliminated from the body and consequently reflects the excretion of the compound.

The most important route of excretion for most compounds is through the kidneys into the urine. Other routes are secretion into the bile, excretion into the expired air from the lungs for volatile and gaseous compounds and secretion into the gastrointestinal tract, milk, sweat and other fluids.

URINARY EXCRETION

Excretion into the urine from the bloodstream applies to relatively small, water-soluble molecules; large molecules such as proteins do not pass out through the intact glomerulus and lipid soluble molecules such as bilirubin are reabsorbed from the kidney tubules.

The kidneys receive approximately 25 per cent of the cardiac output of blood and so they are exposed to and filter out a significant proportion of foreign compounds. Excretion into the urine involves one of three mechanisms: **filtration** from the blood through the pores in the glomerulus; **diffusion** from the bloodstream into the tubules; and **active transport** into the tubular fluid.

The structure of the kidney facilitates the elimination of compounds from the bloodstream (Figure 2.12). The basic unit of the kidney, the **nephron**, allows most small molecules to pass out of the blood in the glomerulus into

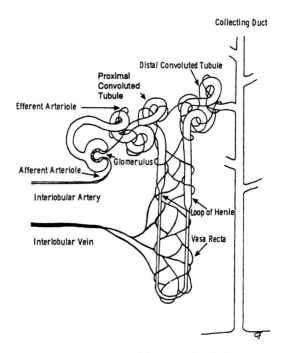

FIGURE 2.12 *Structure of the mammalian kidney. From Timbrell, J. A.,* Principles of Biochemical Toxicology, *Taylor & Francis, London, 2000.*

the tubular ultrafiltrate aided by large pores in the capillaries and the pressure of the blood. Lipid-soluble molecules will passively diffuse out of the blood provided there is a concentration gradient. However, if such compounds are not ionized at the pH of the tubular fluid, they may be reabsorbed from the tubule by passive diffusion back into the blood as it flows through the vessels surrounding the tubule because there will be a concentration gradient in the direction tubule → blood. Water-soluble molecules which are ionized at the pH of the tubular fluid will not be reabsorbed by passive diffusion and will pass out into the urine.

Certain molecules, such as **p-aminohippuric acid**, a metabolite of p-aminobenzoic acid are actively transported from the bloodstream into the tubules by a specific anion transport system.

Passive diffusion of compounds into the tubules is *proportional* to the concentration in the bloodstream, so the greater the amount in the blood the greater will be the rate of elimination. However, when excretion is mediated via **active transport** or **facilitated diffusion**, which involves the use of specific carriers, the rate of elimination is *constant* and the carrier molecules may become **saturated** by large amounts of compound. This may have important **toxicological consequences**. As the dose of a compound is increased, the plasma level will increase. If excretion is via passive diffusion, the rate of excretion will increase as this is proportional to the plasma concentration. If excretion is via active transport, however, increasing the dose may lead to saturation of renal elimination and a toxic level of compound in the plasma and tissues may be reached. This is the case with **ethanol** where continuous intake leads to ever increasing plasma levels accompanied by the well-known effects on the central nervous system.

Another factor which may affect excretion is **binding to plasma proteins**. This may reduce excretion via passive diffusion especially if binding is tight and extensive as only the free portion will be able to passively diffuse into the tubule. Protein binding does not affect active transport however and a compound such as p-aminohippuric acid which is 90 per cent bound to plasma proteins is cleared in the first pass of blood through the kidney.

One of the factors which affects excretion is the **urinary pH**. If the metabolite excreted into the urine is ionizable it may become ionized when it enters the tubular fluid. For example, an acidic drug such as **phenobarbital** is ionized at alkaline urinary pH and a basic drug such as **amphetamine** is ionized at an acidic urinary pH. This factor is utilized in the treatment of poisoning by barbiturates **and aspirin (see below, page 77)**. The pH of urine may be affected by diet; high protein diet for instance causes urine to become more acid. The rate of urine flow from the kidney into the bladder is also a factor in the excretion of foreign compounds; high fluid intake, and therefore production of copious urine, will tend to facilitate excretion.

BILIARY EXCRETION

Excretion into the bile is an important route for certain foreign compounds, especially large **polar** substances. Indeed, it may indeed be the predominant route of elimination. Bile is secreted in the liver by the **hepatocytes** into the **canaliculi** and it flows into the bile duct and eventually into the intestine (Figure 2.13). Consequently compounds which are excreted into the bile are usually eliminated in the faeces. **Molecular weight** is an important factor in biliary excretion as can be seen from Table 2.1 and so for polar compounds with a molecular weight of **300** or so, such as **glutathione conjugates**, biliary excretion can be a major route of excretion. Excretion into the bile is an active process and there are **three specific transport systems**, one for neutral compounds, one for anions and one for cations.

As with renal excretion via active transport, biliary excretion may be saturated and this may lead to an increasing concentration of compound in the liver. For example, the drug **furosemide** was found to cause hepatic damage in mice due to saturation of the biliary excretion route which caused an increase in its concentration in the liver.

Another consequence of biliary excretion is that the compound comes into contact with the **gut microflora**. The bacteria may metabolize the compound and convert it into a more lipid-soluble substance which can be reabsorbed from the intestine into the portal venous blood supply and so return to the liver. This may lead to a cycling of the compound

TABLE 2.1 *Effect of molecular weight on the route of excretion of biphenyls by the rat*

Compound	Molecular weight	% Total excretion	
		Urine	Faeces
Biphenyl	154	80	20
4-Monochlorobiphenyl	188	50	50
4,4'-Dichlorobiphenyl	223	34	66
2,4,5,2',5'-Pentachlorobiphenyl	326	11	89
2,3,6,2',3',6'-Hexachlorobiphenyl	361	1	99

Source: H. B. Matthews (1980), *Introduction to Biochemical Toxicology*, Hodgson and Guthrie (Eds) (New York: Elsevier-North Holland)

known as **enterohepatic recirculation** which may increase the toxicity (Figure 2.13). If the compound is taken orally, and therefore is transported directly to the liver and is extensively excreted into the bile, it may be that none of the parent compound ever reaches the systemic circulation. Alternatively, the gut microflora may metabolize the compound to a more toxic metabolite which could be reabsorbed and cause a systemic toxic effect. Compounds taken orally may also come directly into contact with the gut bacteria. For example, the naturally occurring glycoside cycasin is hydrolyzed to the potent carcinogen **methylazoxymethanol** by the gut bacteria when it is ingested orally.

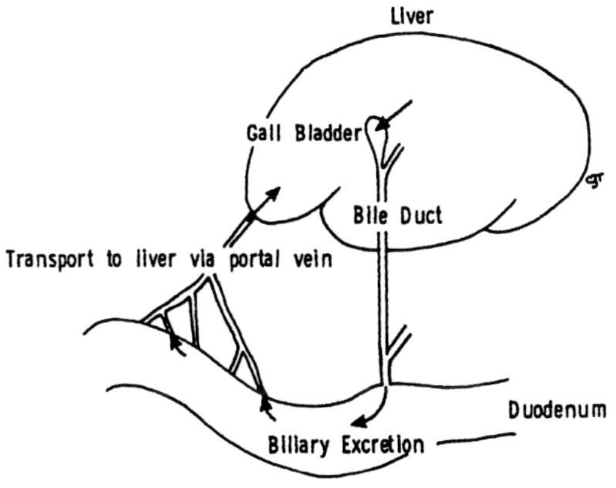

Biliary excretion, therefore, may:

1 **increase the half-life** of the compound;

2 lead to the production of **toxic metabolites** in the gastrointestinal tract;

3 increase hepatic exposure via the **enterohepatic recirculation**;

4 be **saturated** and lead to hepatic damage.

The importance of biliary excretion in the toxicity of compounds can be seen from Table 2.2 which shows that ligation of the bile duct increases the toxicity of certain chemicals many times.

FIGURE 2.13 *Biliary excretion route for foreign compounds.*
From Timbrell, J. A., Principles of Biochemical Toxicology, *Taylor & Francis, London, 2000.*

EXCRETION VIA THE LUNGS

The lungs are an important route of excretion for **volatile** compounds and **gaseous** metabolites of foreign compounds. For example, about 50–60 per cent of a dose of the aromatic hydrocarbon **benzene** is eliminated in the expired air. Excretion is by passive diffusion from the blood into the alveolus assisted by

TABLE 2.2 *Effect of bile duct ligation (BDL) on the toxicity of certain compounds*

Compound	LD$_{50}$; mg/kg		
	Sham operation	BDL	Sham:BDL ratio
Amitryptiline	100	100	1
Diethylstilboestrol	100	0.75	130
Digoxin	11	2.6	4.2
Indocyanine Green	700	130	5.4
Pentobarbital	110	130	0.8

Source: C. D. Klaassen (1974), *Toxicology and Applied Pharmacology,* **24**, 37.

the concentration gradient. This is a very efficient route of excretion for lipid-soluble compounds as the capillary and **alveolar membranes** are **thin** and in very close proximity to allow for the normal gaseous exchange involved in breathing. There will be a continuous concentration gradient between the blood and air in the alveolus because of the rapid removal of the gas or vapour from the lungs and the rapid blood flow to the lungs. This may be a very important factor in the treatment of poisoning by such gases as the highly toxic **carbon monoxide**. Compounds may also be metabolized to volatile metabolites such as carbon dioxide for example.

OTHER ROUTES OF EXCRETION

Excretion into **breast milk** can be a very important route for certain types of compounds especially lipid-soluble compounds. Clearly new born animals will be specifically at risk from toxic compounds excreted into milk. For example nursing mothers exposed to **DDT** secrete it into their milk and the infant may receive a greater dose, on a weight basis, than the mother. Foreign compounds may be secreted into other body fluids such as **sweat**, **tears** or **semen** and certain compounds may be secreted into the **stomach** or **saliva**.

Summary and learning objectives

In this chapter you will have read about *three* of the *four phases* of disposition of a chemical in a biological system: the *absorption* through membranes into the system, the *distribution* throughout the system and the *excretion* and elimination from the system. In the next chapter you will learn about the metabolic fate of chemicals, which is the fourth phase.

All three phases of disposition require the chemical to cross *biological membranes*. Membranes consist of phospholipid bilayers with proteins of various types interspersed. Depending on the chemical structure and its physico-chemical characteristics this will occur by one of a number of processes: *filtration* through pores (small molecules), *passive diffusion* (most foreign chemicals if lipid soluble), *active transport* (chemicals similar to endogenous substances such as amino acids), *facilitated diffusion* (similar chemicals to active transport), **phago/pinocytosis** (large molecules and particles).

Passive diffusion is the most important means of transport of foreign chemicals across biological membranes. It depends on three important factors that together form the *pH partition theory*: the chemical must form a *concentration gradient*, be *lipid soluble* (measured as partition coefficient) and be *non-ionized*. The degree of ionization can be calculated using the *Henderson Hasselbach* equation.

Ficks Law defines the rate of diffusion through membranes and relates it to surface area and the concentration gradient.

Active transport and facilitated diffusion require *carrier proteins* and so can be *saturated* and may undergo *competitive inhibition*. Active transport also requires *energy*.

Absorption occurs from three main sites: *skin* (large surface area, poorly vascularized, not readily permeable); *gastrointestinal tract* (major site, well vascularized, variable pH, large surface area, transport processes, food, gut bacteria), *lungs* (very large surface area, very well vascularized, readily permeable). Also chemicals (e.g. drugs) may be administered by direct injection (i.p., i.m., s.c., i.v.). The result of the absorptive phase is that the compound enters the blood. Absorption from the gastrointestinal tract may result in *first pass metabolism* occurring in the gut wall or liver.

Distribution is the phase in which the compound is carried to the tissues by blood or lymph.

The *plasma level* reflects the concentration at the *target site* and is governed by distribution. It is a vitally important piece of information for the toxicologist. Distribution may be limited by *binding* to plasma proteins. This binding, which is usually non-covalent (ionic, hydrophobic, hydrogen, Van der Waals bonding), may be saturated or be subject to displacement by other compounds allowing threshold effects. The blood level of a chemical can be used to derive *kinetic* parameters such as *half-life*, *area under the curve* (AUC) and *volume of distribution*. Chemicals may be sequestered and *accumulate* in tissue compartments (e.g. adipose tissue) depending on

physico-chemical characteristics such as lipid solubility.

Excretion is the elimination of a chemical from the organism via the urine, bile or expired air. Excretion via the kidney into the *urine* is the major route involving filtration through the glomerulus and passive diffusion, filtration or active transport from the blood into the nephron. Extent of *biliary excretion* is influenced by molecular weight and may result in *enterohepatic recirculation*. Exhalation from the *lungs* involves passive diffusion.

Chemicals may accumulate after repeated exposure if the frequency of dosing is shorter than the half-life or elimination (metabolism or excretion) is saturated.

Questions

Q1. Choose one answer which you think is the most appropriate.
The oil/water partition coefficient of a chemical is an indication of:

    a carcinogenicity
    b long half-life
    c potential to bioaccumulate
    d low apparent volume of distribution
    e chronic toxicity.

Q2. Choose one answer which you think is the most appropriate.
The absorption of which of the following is facilitated by the prevailing pH in the stomach:

    a weak organic bases
    b strong acids
    c weak organic acids
    d strong bases
    e none of the above.

Q3. Choose one answer which you think is the most appropriate.
The parameter 'volume of distribution'

(V_D) may be determined for a chemical *in vivo*. Is it:

a   equal to the water solubility of the chemical

b   sometimes larger than the total body volume

c   equal to the volume of total body water

d   smaller than the total body water if highly bound in tissues

e   none of the above.

Q4.   Choose one answer which you think is the most appropriate.
The half-life of a drug in the blood is determined by:

a   the metabolism of the compound

b   the volume of distribution

c   plasma protein binding

d   absorption of the drug

e   urinary pH

f   the total body clearance.

Q5.   Choose one answer which you think is the most appropriate.
The term 'first-pass effect' means which of the following:

a   the drug is excreted unchanged

b   the drug is mostly metabolized by the gastrointestinal tract and/or liver before reaching the systemic circulation

c   the drug is completely absorbed from the gastrointestinal tract

d   the drug is excreted completely and very quickly by the kidneys

e   none of the above.

Questions 6 and 7. Answer (a) if the statement is true and (b) if the statement is false.

Q6.   The absorption of drugs into biological systems by passive diffusion is facilitated by ionization of the compound.

Q7.   Binding of drugs to proteins in the blood involves the formation of covalent bonds.

Questions 8 and 9.

Select A if 1, 2 and 3 are correct
Select B if 1 and 3 are correct
Select C if 2 and 4 are correct
Select D if only 4 is correct
Select E if all four are correct

Q8.   Which features of a chemical will favour accumulation in biological systems?

1   binding to plasma proteins
2   lipophilicity
3   limited volume of distribution
4   resistance to metabolism.

Q9.   When considering the chronic toxicity (but not acute toxicity) of a chemical which of the following must be considered?

1   nature of the chemical
2   half-life in the body
3   dose of the chemical
4   frequency of dosing.

SHORT ANSWER QUESTIONS

Q10.   Write notes on three of the following:

a   volume of distribution
b   binding of drugs to plasma proteins
c   first-phase effect
d   Fick's law of diffusion.

Q11.   Write notes on three of the following:

a   the pH partition theory
b   plasma half-life
c   plasma clearance
d   enterohepatic recirculation.

Bibliography

BRUIN, A. DE (1976) *Biochemical Toxicology of Environmental Agents,* Amsterdam: Elsevier.

CLARK, B. and SMITH, D. A. (1986) *An Introduction to Pharmacokinetics,* 2nd edition, Oxford: Blackwell.

HATHWAY, D. E. (1984) *Molecular Aspects of Toxicology*, London: The Royal Society of Chemistry.

HODGSON, E. and LEVI, P. E. (1987) *A Textbook of Modern Toxicology,* New York: Elsevier.

HODGSON, E. and LEVI, P. E. (Eds) (1994) *Introduction to Biochemical Toxicology,* Norwalk, Connecticut: Appleton & Lange.

MEDINSKY, M. A. and KLAASSEN, C. D. (1996) Toxicokinetics, Chapter 7, in *Casarett and Doull's Toxicology. The Basic Science of Poisons*, C. D. Klaassen (Ed.) 5th edition, New York: McGraw Hill.

PRATT, W. B. and TAYLOR, P. (Eds) (1990) *Principles of Drug Action: The Basis of Pharmacology,* 3rd edition, New York: Churchill Livingstone.

RENWICK, A. G. (1999) Toxicokinetics, Chapter 4, in *General and Applied Toxicology*, Ballantyne, B., Marrs, T. and Syversen, T. M. (Eds) 2nd edition, Basingstoke: Macmillan.

ROZMAN, K. K. and KLAASSEN, C. D. (1996) Absorption, distribution and excretion of toxicants, Chapter 5, in *Casarett and Doull's Toxicology: The Basic Science of Poisons*, Klaassen, C. D. (Ed.), New York: McGraw-Hill.

TIMBRELL, J. A. (2000) *Principles of Biochemical Toxicology*, 3rd edition, London: Taylor & Francis Ltd. Covers mechanistic and metabolic aspects of toxicology in detail with many examples.

ZBINDEN, G. (1988) Biopharmaceutical studies, a key to better toxicology, *Xenobiotica*, **18**, suppl. 1, 9.

Metabolism of foreign compounds

Chapter outline

From this chapter you will learn about the metabolic fate of chemicals in biological systems and the importance to toxicity:

- The overall purpose of metabolism

- The consequences of metabolism

- Phase 1 reactions – cytochrome P450 and its role in oxidation reactions

- Phase 1 reactions – types of oxidation, reduction and hydrolysis reactions

- Phase 2 reactions – conjugation with glucuronic acid, sulphate, glutathione, amino acids and acetyl groups

- Toxication and detoxication reactions

- Factors affecting toxic responses: species, strain, sex, genetic factors, enzyme induction and inhibition

As we have seen, foreign compounds absorbed into a biological system by passive diffusion are generally lipid soluble and consequently not ideally suited for excretion. For example, very lipophilic substances such as **DDT** (Figure 8.1) and the **polychlorinated biphenyls** are very poorly excreted and hence remain in the animal's body for many years.

After a foreign compound has been absorbed into a biological system it may undergo metabolism (also known as **biotransformation**). The metabolic fate of the compound can have an important bearing on its toxic potential, disposition in the body and its excretion. The products of metabolism are usually more water soluble than the original compound. Indeed, in animals biotransformation seems directed at increasing water solubility and hence excretion. Facilitating the excretion of a compound means that its **biological half-life** is *reduced* and hence its potential **toxicity** is kept to a *minimum*. Metabolism may

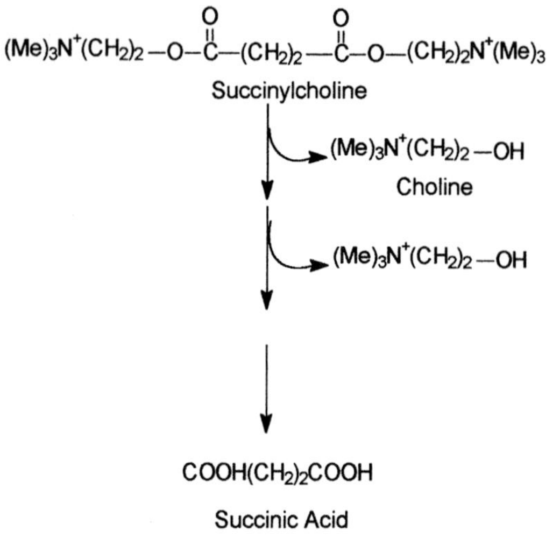

$(Me)_3N^+(CH_2)_2-O-\overset{\displaystyle O}{\overset{\|}{C}}-(CH_2)_2-\overset{\displaystyle O}{\overset{\|}{C}}-O-(CH_2)_2N^+(Me)_3$

Succinylcholine

$\longrightarrow (Me)_3N^+(CH_2)_2-OH$

Choline

$\longrightarrow (Me)_3N^+(CH_2)_2-OH$

$COOH(CH_2)_2COOH$

Succinic Acid

FIGURE 3.1 *Hydrolysis of the drug succinylcholine.*
From Timbrell, J. A., Principles of Biochemical
Toxicology, *Taylor & Francis, London, 2000.*

also directly affect the biological activity of a foreign compound. For example, the drug **suc-cinylcholine** causes muscle relaxation, but its action only lasts a few minutes because metabolism cleaves the molecule to yield inactive products (Figure 3.1). However, in some cases metabolism increases the toxicity of a compound as we shall discuss later in this book. There are numerous examples of this but a well-known one is **ethylene glycol** which is metabolized to oxalic acid, partly responsible for the toxicity (Figure 3.2).

Metabolism, therefore, is an extremely important phase of disposition as it may have a major effect on the **biological activity** of that compound, generally by *increasing* **polarity** and so water **solubility** and thereby *increasing* excretion. For example, the analgesic drug **paracetamol** (discussed in Chapter 5) has a **renal clearance** value of 12 ml min^{-1}, whereas one of its major metabolites, the sulphate conjugate, is cleared at the rate of 170 ml min^{-1}.

Therefore, in summary, metabolism leads to:

1 transformation of the molecule into a **more polar metabolite**;

2 possible **increase** in **molecular weight and size**;

3 **facilitation** of **excretion** and so **elimination** from the organism.

The consequences of these changes are:

a the **half-life** of the compound is *decreased*;

b the **exposure time** is *shortened*;

c the possibility of **accumulation** is *reduced*;

d a probable *change* in biological activity;

e a *change* in the **duration of the biological activity**.

Sometimes metabolism may decrease water solubility and so reduce excretion. For example, **acetylation** *decreases* the solubility of **sulpho-namides** in urine and may lead to crystallization in the kidney tubules causing necrosis of the tissue.

Metabolism can be simply divided into two phases: **phase 1** and **phase 2**. Phase 1 is the alteration of the original foreign molecule so as to add on a functional group which can then be conjugated in phase 2. This can best be understood by examining the example in Figure 3.3. The foreign molecule is **benzene**, a

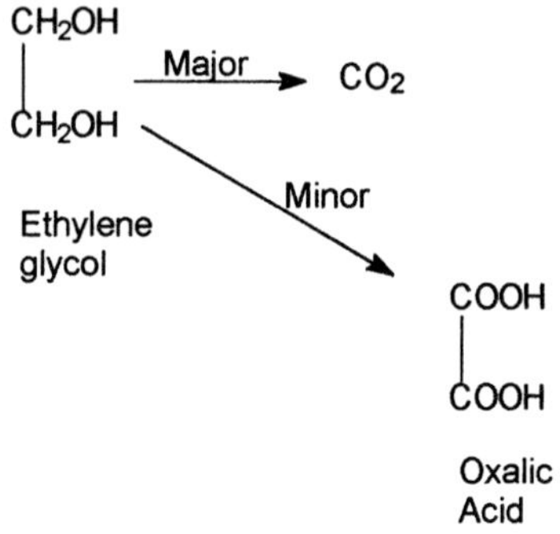

CH$_2$OH
|
CH$_2$OH   — Major →   CO$_2$

Ethylene glycol   Minor

COOH
|
COOH

Oxalic Acid

FIGURE 3.2 *Metabolism of ethylene glycol.*
From Timbrell, J. A., Principles of Biochemical
Toxicology, *Taylor & Francis, London, 2000.*

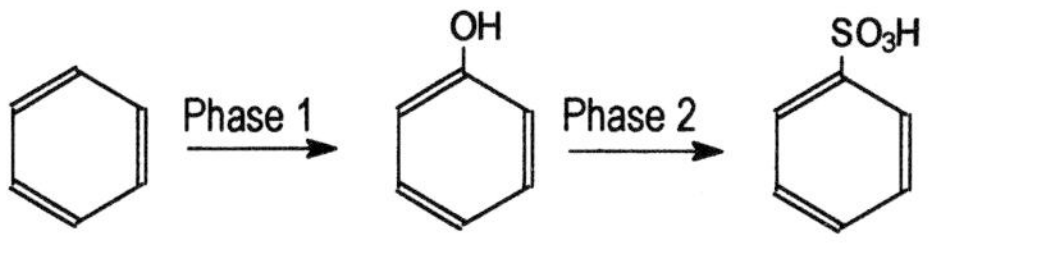

FIGURE 3.3 *Metabolism of benzene.*
From Timbrell, J. A., Principles of Biochemical
Toxicology, *Taylor & Francis, London, 2000.*

highly lipophilic molecule which is not readily excreted from the animal except in the **expired air** as it is volatile. Phase 1 metabolism converts benzene into a variety of metabolites, but the major one is **phenol**. The insertion of a **hydroxyl** group allows a phase 2 conjugation reaction to take place with the polar **sulphate** group being added. Phenyl sulphate, the final metabolite, is very water soluble and is readily excreted in the urine.

Most biotransformations can be divided into phase 1 and phase 2 reactions, although some foreign molecules already possess functional groups suitable for phase 2 reactions, such as phenol for example. The products of phase 2 biotransformations may be further metabolized in what is sometimes termed **phase 3 reactions**.

Metabolism is usually catalyzed by enzymes and these are usually, but not always, found most abundantly in the liver in animals. The reason for this location is that most foreign compounds enter the body via the gastrointestinal tract and the portal blood supply goes directly to the liver (Figure 2.7). However, it is important to remember that **(1)** the enzymes involved with the metabolism of foreign compounds may be found in many other tissues as well as the liver; **(2)** the enzymes may be localized in one particular cell type in an organ; and **(3)** the enzymes are not always specific for foreign compounds and may have a major role in normal endogenous metabolism.

The **enzymes** involved in biotransformation also have a particular subcellular localization:

many are found in the **endoplasmic reticulum**. Some are located in the cytosol and a few are found in other organelles such as the mitochondrion. The various types of metabolic reactions are shown in Table 3.1. For more information on the metabolism of foreign compounds the reader should consult the more detailed texts indicated in the bibliography.

PHASE 1 REACTIONS

Oxidation reactions

The majority of these reactions are catalyzed by one enzyme system, the **cytochrome P450 mono-oxygenase** system which is located in the smooth endoplasmic reticulum of the cell, isolated as the so-called microsomal fraction obtained by cell fractionation. The liver has the highest concentration of this enzyme although it can be found in most, if not all tissues. The reactions catalyzed also require **NADPH**, molecular **oxygen** and **magnesium**, and the overall reaction is shown below:

$$SH + O_2 + NADPH + H^+ \rightarrow SOH + H_2O + NADP^+$$

where S is the substrate.

The sequence of metabolic reactions is shown in Figure 3.4 and involves four distinct steps:

TABLE 3.1 *The major biotransformation reactions*

Phase I	Phase 2
Oxidation	Sulphation
Reduction	Glucuronidation
Hydrolysis	Glutathione conjugation
Hydration	Acetylation
Dehalogenation	Amino acid conjugation

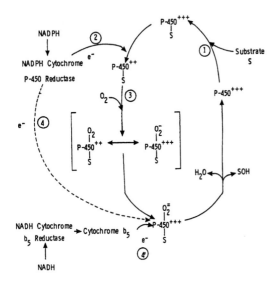

FIGURE 3.4   *The cytochrome P450 mono-oxygenase system which catalyzes the phase 1 metabolism of many foreign compounds.*
From Timbrell, J. A., Principles of Biochemical Toxicology, *Taylor & Francis, London, 2000.*

1   addition of **substrate** to the enzyme;

2   donation of an **electron**;

3   addition of **oxygen** and rearrangement;

4   donation of a **second electron** and loss of water.

Cytochrome P450

The cytochrome P450 mono-oxygenase system is actually a collection of isoenzymes (at least forty in humans) based on a haem protein, at the centre of which is an iron atom. The system also requires another enzyme, **NADPH cytochrome P450 reductase**, which donates electrons to the cytochrome P450. Although the enzyme is mainly located in the SER other organelles such as the nucleus also have some activity. There are at least twenty-seven gene families in the cytochrome P450 gene superfamily. The enzyme protein is designated CYP and

there are three families especially involved with the metabolism of xenobiotics, CYP 1, CYP 2 and CYP 3. CYP 4 is responsible for the metabolism of fatty acids but may also be involved in the metabolism of xenobiotics. A number of the isozymes show **genetic polymorphisms** which influence the metabolism of drugs and other chemicals (see later). The proportions of isoenzymes varies between different tissues in the same animal and between different species of animal. There may also be differences between different sexes and other factors such as exposure to xenobiotics which may induce particular isozymes.

Cytochrome P450 carries out about sixty different types of reaction and the isozymes have broad and overlapping substrate specificity.

Although there is a large variety of types of substrate for cytochrome P450, one factor in common is that most are lipophilic. There is indeed a correlation between the metabolism and lipophilicity of chemicals metabolized by the enzyme with the more lipophilic being better substrates.

Cytochrome P450 shows a number of polymorphisms which may affect the metabolism of drugs and other chemicals. Thus there may be considerable differences between individual humans in terms of their ability to metabolize drugs and other chemicals. (See below under genetic factors.) These catalyze different types of oxidation reactions and under certain circumstances catalyze other types of reaction.

Let us look at the major types of oxidation reaction catalyzed by the cytochrome P450 system.

Aromatic hydroxylation, such as occurs with benzene (Figure 3.3) and **aliphatic** hydroxylation such as with **vinyl chloride** (Figure 3.5) involves adding oxygen across a double bond. Hydroxylation of the aliphatic moiety in **propylbenzene** may occur at one of three positions (Figure 3.6). **Alicyclic** and **heterocyclic** rings may also undergo hydroxylation.

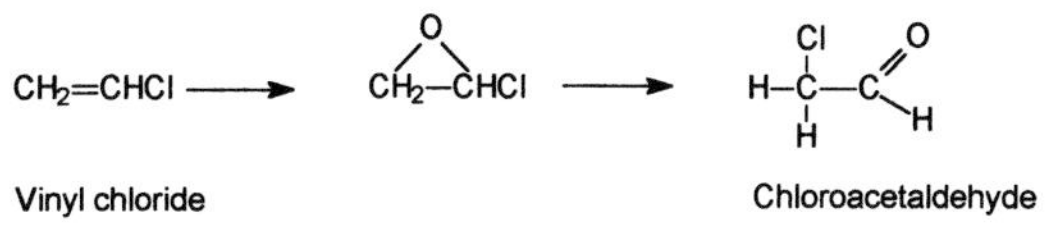

FIGURE 3.5 *Epoxidation of vinyl chloride.*
From Timbrell, J. A., Principles of Biochemical
Toxicology, *Taylor & Francis, London, 2000.*

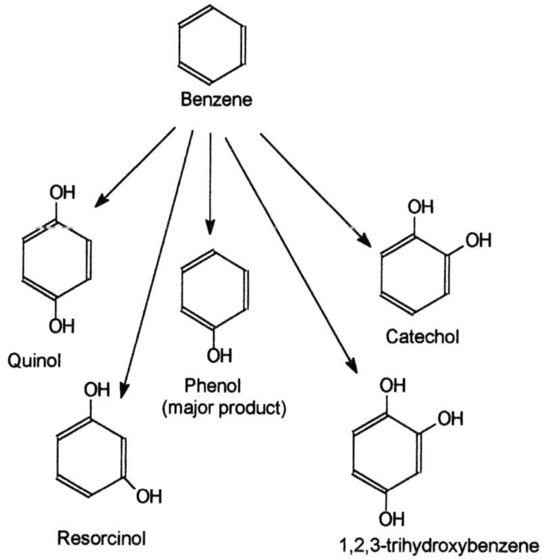

FIGURE 3.6 *Oxidation of n-propylbenzene.*
From Timbrell, J. A., Principles of Biochemical
Toxicology, *Taylor & Francis, London, 2000.*

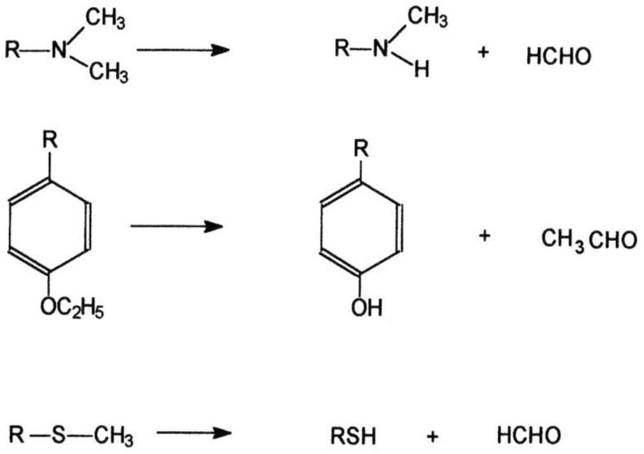

FIGURE 3.7 *Dealkylation reactions.*
From Timbrell, J. A., Principles of Biochemical
Toxicology, *Taylor & Francis, London, 2000.*

Another important group of enzymes which catalyze oxidation reactions for foreign compounds are the **peroxidases**. For example, the toxic solvent benzene, which causes **aplastic anaemia**, is believed to be metabolized by peroxidases in the bone marrow. The drug **hydralazine** is also believed to be metabolized by this enzyme system (see Chapter 5).

Reduction reactions

These reactions may be catalyzed by either microsomal or cytosolic **reductases** and by the **gut bacteria**, which also possess reductases. The most commonly encountered type of reductive reaction is the reduction of **nitro** and **azo** groups such as those present in the food colour **tartrazine** (Figure 3.12). Less common reduction reactions include reduction of

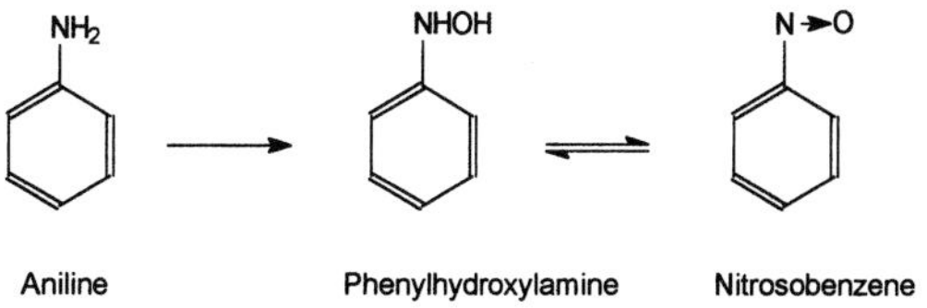

Alkyl groups attached to **N, O or S** atoms may be removed by **dealkylation** reactions which involve oxidation of the alkyl group and then rearrangement and loss as the respective **aldehyde** (Figure 3.7). Nitrogen and sulphur atoms in xenobiotics may be oxidized by the microsomal enzymes (Figure 3.8) and sulphur and halogen atoms may be removed oxidatively (Figures 3.9 and 3.10).

Certain oxidation reactions are catalyzed by other enzymes such as **alcohol dehydrogenase** (Figure 3.11), **xanthine oxidase, microsomal amine oxidase, monoamine** and **diamine oxidases**.

FIGURE 3.8 *N-hydroxylation of an aromatic amino group.*
From Timbrell, J. A., Principles of Biochemical
Toxicology, *Taylor & Francis, London, 2000.*

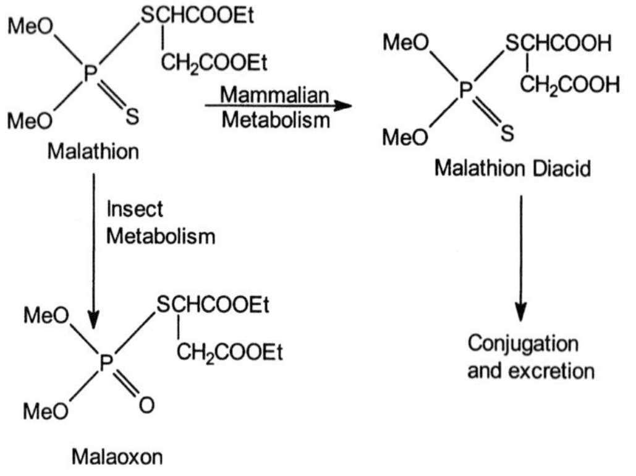

FIGURE 3.9 *Metabolism of the insecticide malathion. From Timbrell, J. A.,* Principles of Biochemical Toxicology, *Taylor & Francis, London, 2000.*

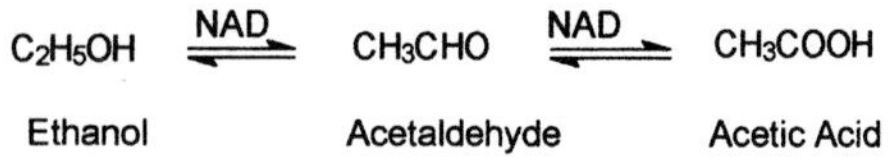

FIGURE 3.11 *Oxidation of the primary alcohol ethanol. From Timbrell, J. A.,* Principles of Biochemical Toxicology, *Taylor & Francis, London, 2000.*

aldehyde and **keto** groups, **epoxides** and **double bonds**.

Reductive dehalogenation, catalyzed by the microsomal enzyme system is an important route of metabolism for anaesthetics such as **halothane** (Figure 3.10) (see Chapter 5).

Reductive dechlorination is involved in the toxicity of **carbon tetrachloride**.

Hydrolysis

Esters and **amides** are hydrolyzed by **esterases** and **amidases** respectively, and there are a number of these enzymes, which are usually found in the cytosol of cells in a variety of tissues. Some are also found in the plasma. Microsomal esterases have also been described. Typical esterase and amidase reactions are shown in Figure 3.13. An example of esterase

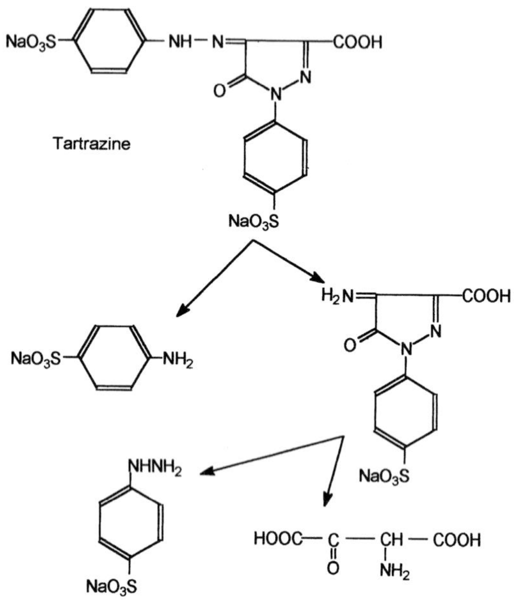

FIGURE 3.12 *Metabolic reduction of the food-colouring agent tartrazine.*

action which is *toxicologically* important is that of the hydrolysis of the drug **succinyl choline**. The very short duration of action of this compound is due to it being very rapidly hydrolyzed in the plasma (see Chapter 5). Amidases have an important role in the toxicity

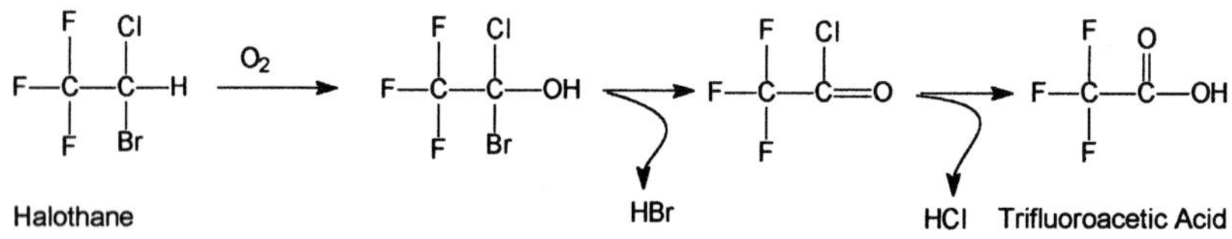

FIGURE 3.10 *The metabolism of the anaesthetic halothane showing the oxidative pathway. The penultimate product, trifluoroacetyl chloride is believed to be the reactive intermediate which acylates liver proteins.*

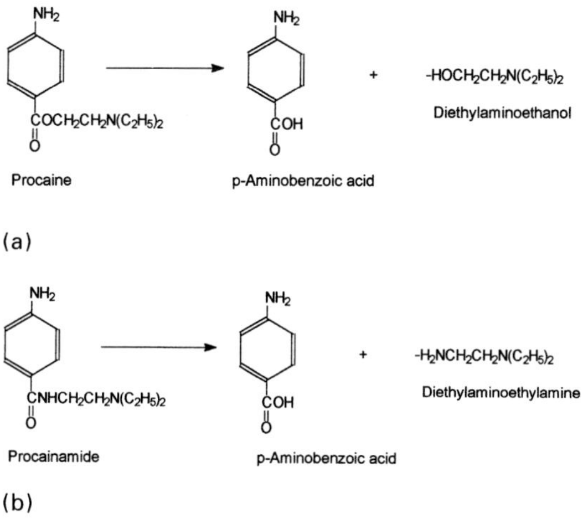

(a)

(b)

FIGURE 3.13 *Hydrolysis of an ester (the drug procaine) and an amide (the drug procainamide). From Timbrell, J. A.,* Principles of Biochemical Toxicology, *Taylor & Francis, London, 2000.*

of the drugs **isoniazid** and **phenacetin**, where hydrolysis is an important step in the metabolic activation.

Hydration

Epoxides, which can be stable metabolic intermediates, may undergo hydration catalyzed by the enzyme **epoxide hydrolase** located in the microsomal fraction. This is usually a *detoxication* reaction as the dihydrodiol products are normally much less chemically reactive than the epoxide.

PHASE 2 REACTIONS

These reactions, also known as **conjugation** reactions, involve the addition of a **polar group** to the foreign molecule. This polar group is either conjugated to an existing group or to one added in a phase 1 reaction, such as a hydroxyl group. The polar group renders the foreign molecule *more* water **soluble** and so more readily cleared from the body and less likely to exert a toxic effect. The groups donated in phase 2 reactions are commonly those involved in intermediary metabolism. Conjugation reactions are considered below.

Sulphation

The addition of the sulphate moiety to a **hydroxyl** group is a major route of conjugation for foreign compounds. It is catalyzed by a cytosolic **sulphotransferase** enzyme and utilizes the coenzyme **phosphoadenosine phosphosulphate**. The product is an ester which is very polar and water soluble. Both aromatic and aliphatic hydroxyl groups may be conjugated with sulphate as may N-hydroxy groups and amino groups (Figure 3.14).

Glucuronidation

Glucuronic acid is a polar and water soluble carbohydrate molecule which may be added to **hydroxyl** groups, **carboxylic acid** groups, **amino** groups and **thiols** (Figure 3.15). This

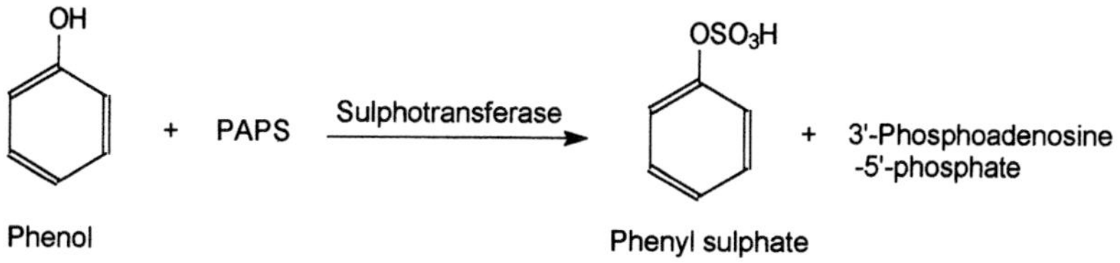

FIGURE 3.14 *Conjugation of a phenol and an aliphatic alcohol with sulphate. PAPS is the sulphate donor, phosphoadenosinephosphosulphate. From Timbrell, J. A.,* Principles of Biochemical Toxicology, *Taylor & Francis, London, 2000.*

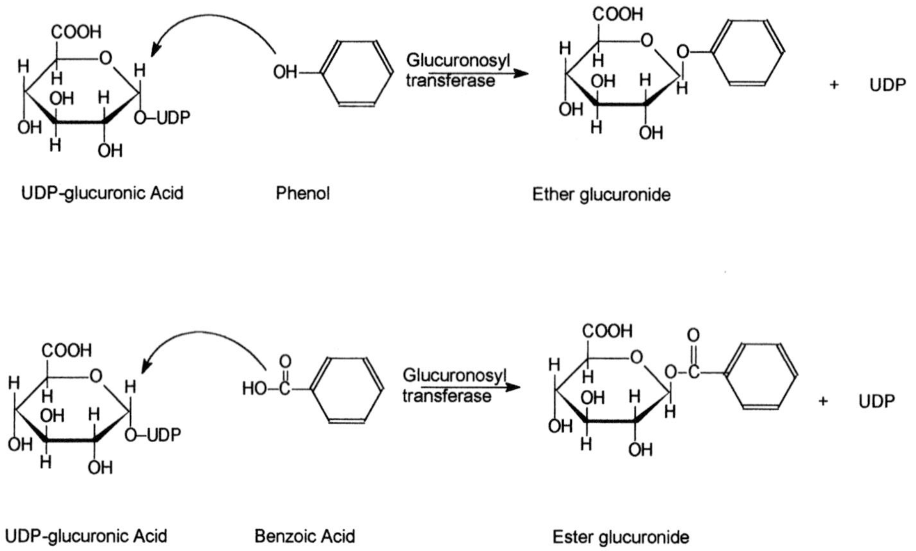

FIGURE 3.15 *Conjugation of a phenol and a carboxylic acid with glucuronic acid.*
From Timbrell, J. A., Principles of Biochemical Toxicology, *Taylor & Francis, London, 2000.*

process is a major route of phase 2 metabolism and utilizes **glucuronosyl transferases**, which are microsomal enzymes, with **uridine diphosphate glucuronic acid** as the cofactor. Other carbohydrates may also be involved in conjugation such as **glucose**, which is utilized by insects to form glucosides. **Ribose** and **xylose** may also be used in conjugation reactions.

Glutathione conjugation

This is a particularly important route of phase 2 metabolism from the *toxicological* point of view as it is often involved in the removal of **reactive intermediates**. Glutathione is a **tripeptide** found in many mammalian tissues, but especially in the liver. It has a major *protective* role in the body as it is a scavenger for reactive compounds of various types, combining at the reactive centre in the molecule and so reducing or abolishing the toxicity. Normally, the **sulphydryl group** of glutathione acts as a **nucleophile** and either displaces another atom or attacks an electrophilic site (Figure 3.16). Consequently glutathione may

react either chemically or in enzyme-catalyzed reactions with a variety of compounds which are either reactive or are electrophilic metabolites produced in phase 1 reactions. The reactions may be catalyzed by one of a group of **glutathione transferases** located in the soluble fraction of the cell. They have been detected also in the microsomal fraction. The substrates include aromatic, heterocyclic, alicyclic and aliphatic **epoxides**, aromatic **halogen** and **nitro** compounds and **unsaturated aliphatic compounds**. The conjugate which results may be either excreted into the bile unchanged or metabolized further, via so-called phase 3 reactions, to yield an N-acetylcysteine conjugate or **mercapturic acid** (Figure 3.16).

Acetylation

This metabolic reaction is unusual in that the product may be *less water soluble* than the parent compound. Substrates for acetylation are aromatic **amino compounds, sulphonamides, hydrazines** and **hydrazides** (Figure 3.17).

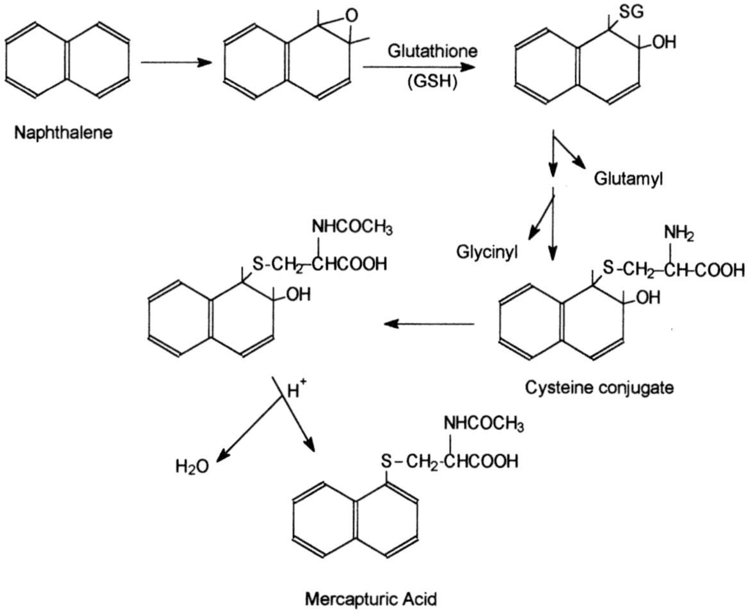

FIGURE 3.16 *Metabolism of naphthalene showing the conjugation of naphthalene epoxide with glutathione and the subsequent formation of a N-acetylcysteine conjugate (mercapturic acid).*
From Timbrell, J. A., Principles of Biochemical Toxicology, *Taylor & Francis, London, 2000.*

The enzymes involved are **acetyltransferases** and are found in the cytosol of cells in the liver, gastric mucosa and white blood cells. The enzymes utilize **acetyl Coenzyme A**

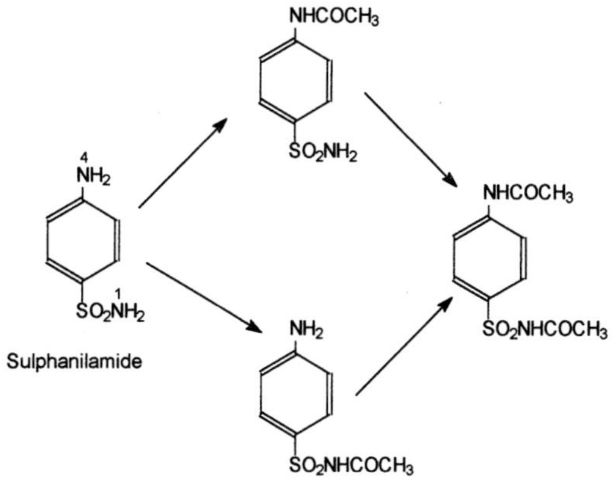

FIGURE 3.17 *The acetylation of the amino and sulphonamido groups of the drug sulphanilamide.*
From Timbrell, J. A., Principles of Biochemical Toxicology, *Taylor & Francis, London, 2000.*

as cofactor. There are **two isoenzymes** in the rabbit which differ markedly in activity and the same is probably true in humans. In both species the possession of a particular isoenzyme is genetically determined and gives rise to two distinct **phenotypes** known as 'rapid' and 'slow' acetylators. This has an important role in the toxicity of certain drugs such as **hydralazine** (see Chapter 5), **isoniazid** and **procainamide**, and these examples illustrate the importance of **genetic factors** in toxicology.

Amino acid conjugation

Foreign **organic acids** may undergo conjugation with amino acids (as well as with glucuronic acid, see above). The particular amino acid utilized depends on the species concerned and, indeed, species within a similar evolutionary group tend to utilize the same amino acid. **Glycine** is the most common amino acid used.

The carboxylic acid group first reacts with Coenzyme A and then with the particular amino acid. The **acylase** enzyme catalyzing the reaction is found in the mitochondria.

Methylation

Hydroxyl, amino and **thiol** groups in molecules may be methylated by one of a series of **methyltransferases**. This occurs particularly with endogenous compounds but xenobiotics may also be substrates. As with acetylation this reaction tends to *decrease* rather than increase **water solubility**.

An important *toxicological* example is the methylation of heavy metals such as **mercury**. This may be carried out by micro-organisms in the environment (see Chapter 9). The importance is that this *changes* the **physico-chemical characteristics** of mercury from a **water-soluble** inorganic ion, to a **lipid-soluble** organic compound. There is also a corresponding *change* in the **toxicity** of mercury with mercuric ion being toxic to the **kidney** in contrast to organomercury which is toxic to the **nervous system**.

There are other reactions that a foreign molecule may undergo but the interested reader should consult one of the texts or reviews given in the bibliography. One important point to remember, however, is that although a molecule is *foreign* to a living organism, it may still be a substrate for an enzyme involved in *normal* metabolic pathways, provided its chemical structure is appropriate, and so this widens the scope of potential metabolic reactions. Foreign compounds can be metabolized by a number of different enzymes simultaneously in the same animal and so there may be many different metabolic routes and metabolites. The balance between these routes can often determine the toxicity of the compound.

TOXICATION VERSUS DETOXICATION

The metabolism of foreign compounds has been termed detoxication because in general it converts these compounds into more water-soluble, readily excreted substances and *decreases* the **toxicity**. However, in some cases the reverse occurs and a metabolite is produced which is *more* **toxic** than the parent compound. A prime example of this is the drug **paracetamol** (acetaminophen) which is discussed in more detail in Chapter 5. However, in this case there are several pathways of metabolism that compete. Consequently, factors that alter the balance between these pathways will alter the eventual toxicity. This *balance* between **toxication** and **detoxication** pathways (Figure 3.18) is very important in toxicology and underlies some of the factors that affect toxicity. These will be discussed later in this chapter.

Factors affecting toxic responses

As already indicated, metabolism is a major factor in determining the toxicity of a com-

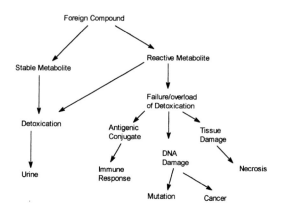

FIGURE 3.18 *An illustration of the ways in which the metabolism of a compound may have a variety of consequences for the organism.*

pound. Factors that affect the disposition will consequently affect toxicity. There are many such factors, which may be either chemical or biological. Chemical factors include the physico-chemical characteristics (**pK$_a$, lipophilicity, size, shape**) and **chirality** (various types of isomers). Biological factors are more numerous and include **species, genetics, diet, age, sex, pathological state**. Many of these factors affect metabolism and so may influence the toxicity of the compound. For example, different isomers may be metabolized differently and hence show different biological activity. In humans, genetic differences may affect metabolism and consequently toxicity. Different species will have different metabolic capabilities and, therefore, may be more or less susceptible to the toxic effects of some compounds. Dietary constituents may influence metabolic pathways or rate of metabolism and, therefore, whether or not a compound is toxic. However, many of these factors will be discussed and highlighted in examples in later chapters and so will not be discussed in detail here.

SPECIES

Species often vary widely in their responses to toxic compounds and this may be extremely important in relation to veterinary medicine, human medicine and environmental toxicology. For example, **drugs** are tested in animals for eventual use in man. If the response in the human animal is very different from that in rats or mice problems may arise when the drug undergoes clinical trials (see Chapter 12).

Similarly, veterinary products may be used on a variety of species and if there are big differences in toxicity this may lead to fatalities or pathological damage in farm animals or pets. For example **cats** have been found to

be particularly susceptible to the toxic effects of paracetamol. This is because **paracetamol** detoxication by conjugation with glucuronic acid is deficient in the cat which therefore has to rely on sulphate conjugation, which may be easily saturated. Consequently, the cytochrome P450 mediated pathway which produces a toxic metabolite (see below Chapter 5) becomes more significant and the cat suffers liver damage more readily. In the environment very large numbers of widely different species may all be exposed to a pesticide and may react very differently. Indeed this difference in sensitivity is exploited in pesticides. Insecticides, such as **organophosphorus compounds** and **DDT** (see Chapter 8), are much more toxic to insects than to humans and other mammals; in some cases this is due to metabolic differences. For example, the insecticide **malathion** is metabolized by *hydrolysis* in mammals but is *oxidized* in the insect to malaoxon which then binds to and inhibits the enzyme **cholinesterase** (Figures 3.9 and 8.4; see also Chapter 8).

One of the problems associated with species differences in metabolism is the use of animals for the safety evaluation of drugs and other chemicals. The testing of such compounds of necessity has to be carried out in animals prior to human exposure but choosing the 'right' animal model may be difficult, especially because human metabolism of the chemical may be very different from the commonly used experimental species. Also, of course, species may vary in their response to chemicals, although this is probably less common than metabolic differences between species. (See also Chapter 12.)

There are very many species differences in metabolism and it is beyond the scope of this book to discuss them in detail. The interested reader is recommended to consult the bibliography at the end of this chapter.

STRAIN OF ANIMAL

Just as different species may vary in their response to toxic compounds and in the way they metabolize them, different inbred strains of the same animal may also show variation. For example, different strains of mice vary widely in their ability to metabolize **barbiturates** and consequently the magnitude of the pharmacological effect varies between the strains (Table 3.2).

SEX

Males and females can also differ in their responses due to **metabolic** and **hormonal differences**. Males in some species metabolize compounds *more rapidly* than females, although this difference is not found in all species. As well as metabolic differences there are examples of sex differences in *routes* of excretion which underlie differences in *susceptibility*. For example, **dinitrotoluene**-induced hepatic tumours occur predominantly in males due to the differences in the route of excretion. Biliary excretion of a glucuronide conjugate is favoured in males while urinary excretion predominates in females.

TABLE 3.2 *Strain differences in the duration of action of hexobarbital in mice*

Strain	Sleeping time
A /NL	48 ± 4
BALB /cAnN	41 ± 2
C57L /HeN	33 ± 3
C3HfB /HeN	22 ± 3
SWR /HeN	18 ± 4
Swiss (non-inbred)	43 ± 15

Source: G. E. Jay (1955), *Proceedings of the Society of Experimental Biology and Medicine*, 90, 378

The glucuronide conjugate is broken down in the intestine by gut bacteria and the products are reabsorbed, causing the hepatic tumours. The difference in susceptibility to **chloroform**-induced kidney damage between male and female mice is an example of a sex difference which has a metabolic basis and hormonal basis. The male mice are more susceptible but this difference can be removed by castration and restored by **androgens**. It may be that **testosterone** is influencing the microsomal enzyme-mediated *metabolism* of chloroform to give greater metabolism in males.

GENETIC FACTORS AND HUMAN VARIABILITY IN RESPONSE

Genetic variation is particularly important in the **human** population which is genetically mixed. There are now many examples of **toxic drug reactions** which occur in individuals due to a genetic defect or genetic difference in metabolism. The best known example in man is that of the **acetylator phenotype** where the acetylation reaction (see page 46) shows genetic variations which are due to mutations giving rise to mutant alleles. This results in rapid and slow acetylators where the latter have *less functional* **acetyltransferase enzyme**. This is an important factor in a number of adverse drug reactions including the **hydralazine-induced lupus syndrome** discussed in Chapter 4, **procainamide**-induced lupus syndrome, **isoniazid**-induced liver damage and **isoniazid**-induced peripheral neuropathy.

The first genetic polymorphism of cytochrome P450 to be discovered and perhaps the most well characterized is that affecting **CYP2D6** which catalyses the metabolism of the drugs **debrisoquine**, **bufuralol** and **sparteine**, for example. (See also below Chapter 5 under debrisoquine.) There are two phenotypes resulting from this polymorphism, known as poor metabolizers and extensive metabolizers. Poor metabolizers are individuals who have reduced metabolic activity towards certain substrates due to almost the complete absence of functional cytochrome P4502D6 as a result of one of a number of mutations. These mutations produce abnormal mRNA, and hence abnormal enzyme protein. Poor metabolizers may suffer increased toxicity from some drugs such as **penicillamine**, which may cause skin rashes, and **phenformin**, which may be associated with lactic acidosis. The poor metabolizer phenotype occurs in approximately 5–10 per cent of the white Caucasian population. A similar genetic polymorphism occurs with cytochrome **P4502C**, which is particularly common in the **Japanese** population.

Other enzymes involved in drug metabolism may also be subject to genetic variation such as **alcohol dehydrogenase** and **esterases**. These variations may also underlie toxic or exaggerated responses. For example, increased sensitivity to **alcohol** may result from reduced metabolism in some individuals such as **North American Indians**. This is caused by a variant of alcohol dehydrogenase that metabolizes alcohol at a slower rate in certain individuals. There are indeed a number of variants of alcohol dehydrogenase that occur in different ethnic groups and some are associated with particular reactions to alcohol exposure.

Similarly **esterases** show a number of polymorphisms. For example, the metabolism of **succinylcholine (suxamethonium)**, a muscle relaxant drug, can show considerable variation between human individuals. This in turn affects the duration of action of the drug. Thus, in most individuals, muscle relaxation after succinyl choline lasts a matter of minutes, whereas in a few individuals with a particular isoform of pseudocholinesterase, metabolism is reduced and the relaxation can last for an hour or more and may become life threatening.

Toxic responses to foreign chemicals may show large variation between human subjects and some of this variation can be ascribed to the factors mentioned. As well as genetically determined metabolic differences, there may be genetic differences in a receptor or in an immunological parameter giving rise to variation in toxicological and pharmacological responses to drugs and other foreign compounds. Several examples will be discussed later in this book. In some cases, however, rare idiosyncratic reactions of unknown origin may occur and in other cases a combination of factors may be necessary for a toxic reaction to occur (see Chapter 5; hydralazine). Unfortunately, much of the variability seen in humans is not encountered in inbred experimental animals and consequently rare but severe and life-threatening toxic reactions may not be encountered in toxicity studies in animals and may only become known after very large numbers of humans have been exposed to the particular chemical.

ENVIRONMENTAL FACTORS

Another factor which affects the human population is the environment, in particular the other chemical substances to which people are exposed. Thus, chemicals in the diet, air or water may all influence the toxic response to another chemical. Unlike experimental animals, humans may be under medication with several drugs when exposure to an industrial chemical occurs, for instance. These drugs can influence the way in which the body reacts to the chemical. The intake of one drug may affect the response to another. Repeated exposure of animals to chemicals may increase the *in vivo* activity of enzymes involved with the metabolism of xenobiotics. In some cases this may be the enzymes that are responsible for metabolism of the chemical itself. This phenomenon is known as enzyme induction and is due to increased amounts of the enzyme, possibly as a result of increased synthesis. There are a number of enzymes involved with xenobiotic metabolism which may be induced but possibly the most important is cytochrome P450. Phase 2 enzymes may also be induced such as glucuronosyl transferase. The **induction** of these enzymes can lead to either increased or decreased toxicity of a compound. Therefore exposure to such substances, which might be drugs or environmental chemicals, can have a significant effect on the toxicity of another substance such as a co-administered drug or another environmental chemical. For example, overdoses of **paracetamol** are more likely to cause serious liver damage if the victim is also exposed to large amounts of **alcohol** or **barbiturate**, both of which *induce* drug metabolizing enzymes and thereby **increase** the *in vivo* activity.

Enzyme induction may also alter endogenous metabolic pathways such as the synthesis of steroids.

Conversely, some chemicals can act as enzyme inhibitors and thereby alter the metabolism of other chemicals and possibly increase their toxicity. Enzyme inhibitors could be drugs or industrial chemicals. Unlike enzyme inducers, **inhibitors** usually act after a single exposure. Both enzyme inducers and inhibitors may be natural constituents of the diet or regularly used drugs such as alcohol or tobacco. **Alcohol** is especially important as an enzyme inducer in relation to drug use and abuse.

A recent example of a naturally occurring inhibitor is a flavonoid found in **grapefruit juice** which is a potent inhibitor of cytochrome **P450 3A4**.

Compounds which inhibit metabolic pathways by blocking particular enzymes may also be factors in toxic responses. For example, workers exposed to the solvent **dimethylformamide** seem more likely to suffer **alcohol-**induced flushes than those not exposed, possibly due to the *inhibition* of alcohol metabolism. The diet contains many substances which may influence the enzymes of drug metabolism such as the microsomal enzyme inducer *β*-**naphthoflavone** found in certain vegetables. **Cigarette smoking** and **alcohol** intake also are known to affect drug metabolism and pharmacological and toxicological responses.

Although enzyme induction and inhibition can be important with regard to the disposition and toxicity of environmental chemicals, it is probably more often a significant problem with drugs. This is because drugs are commonly administered together, possibly for extended periods and at higher concentrations than those of environmental chemicals to which we are exposed.

PATHOLOGICAL STATE

The influence of disease states on metabolism and toxicity has not been well explored. Diseases of the **liver** will clearly affect metabolism but different liver diseases can influence metabolism differently. Disease states such as **influenza** are also known to affect drug metabolizing enzymes, possibly via the production of **interferon**.

Summary and learning objectives

This chapter has been concerned with *metabolism or biotransformation* of chemicals, the enzyme catalyzed conversion of the molecule into products with altered physico-chemical and biological properties. These are usually *more water soluble*, *less lipid soluble* and often of greater molecular weight. Therefore the **consequences of metabolism** are increased excretion, shortened half-life and reduced accumulation and exposure of the biological system to potentially toxic compounds. Metabolism of a chemical is determined by its structure, properties and available enzymes. It can be divided into two phases: **phase 1** predominantly **oxidation** but also **reduction** and **hydrolysis**; **phase 2, conjugation**. Phase 1 results in the generation of a functional group; phase 2 involves addition of an endogenous moiety to that functional group to increase water solubility. The most important enzyme involved in phase 1 oxidation reactions is the **cytochrome P450 system** (27 gene families; 3–4 involved with chemical metabolism), of which there are many isoforms and it is located in the smooth endoplasmic reticulum. Some of the isoforms show genetic polymorphisms. Other oxidative enzymes include alcohol dehydrogenase, xanthine oxidase, microsomal amine oxidase, monoamine and diamine oxidases and peroxidases. **Reduction** is commonly catalyzed by reductases (azo- and nitro-) in gut bacteria. **Hydrolysis** (ester and amide) is catalyzed by esterases. Hydration of epoxides, a detoxication reaction, is catalyzed by a microsomal epoxide hydrolase.

The main phase 2 reactions are addition of **glucuronic acid**, **sulphate**, **glutathione**, **amino acids** and **acetylation** catalyzed by transferases. Glutathione conjugation is an important detoxication reaction.

The **balance** of metabolic pathways may determine whether a compound undergoes **toxication** or **detoxication**.

Metabolism may be affected by chemical, biological and environmental factors. Physicochemical factors such as chirality, size, shape, lipophilicity are important. Biological factors include **species and strain**, **genetic differences in humans**, **age**, **sex**, **disease** and **diet/nutrition**. Species differences are important for drug safety testing and pesticide design. Genetic factors are important in human response. Disease may reduce metabolism. Environmental factors include the influence of other drugs, food constituents or environmental contaminants as **inducers** or **inhibitors**.

Questions

Q1. Choose one answer which you think is the most appropriate.
Metabolism of a foreign chemical will lead to:

   a   accumulation of the chemical in the tissues
   b   increased excretion in urine
   c   decreased toxicity
   d   altered chemical structure
   e   increased toxicity.

Q2. Indicate which of the following statements is true and which is false.
Cytochrome P450 is an enzyme which:

   a   is found in lysosomes
   b   is responsible for the conjugation of drugs
   c   is a central part of the drug metabolizing system
   d   is one of the enzymes in the mitochondrial electron transport chain
   e   c and d are correct.

Q3. Choose one answer which you think is the most appropriate.
Phase 2 metabolism usually involves:

   a   microsomal enzymes
   b   decreasing the polarity of a chemical
   c   increasing the toxicity of compounds
   d   the addition of an endogenous moiety
   e   hydrolysis.

Q4. Indicate which of the following is true and which false:
Glutathione is:

a a protein
b a tripeptide
c an enzyme involved in detoxication
d a substance found in the kidneys
e a vitamin.

Q5. Answer a if the statement is true and b if the statement is false.
Cytochrome P450 mainly catalyses the phase 1 metabolism of chemicals.

Q6. Select A if 1, 2 and 3 are correct
Select B if 1 and 3 are correct
Select C if 2 and 4 are correct
Select D if only 4 is correct
Select E if all four are correct

The microsomal enzyme system is responsible for the metabolism of foreign compounds. Which of the following are essential aspects of this system?

1 magnesium ions
2 the addition of two electrons
3 molecular oxygen
4 the substrate is bound to an iron atom in the active site.

Q7. Indicate which of the following is true and which false:
The acetylator phenotype is:

a not found in dogs
b found exclusively in Orientals
c responsible for the toxicity of amines
d an inherited trait affecting a particular metabolic reaction
e associated with the HLA type.

Q8. Choose one answer which you think is the most appropriate.
The phenomenon of enzyme induction involves:

a an increase in the synthesis of the enzyme
b an increase in the activity of the enzyme
c an increase in liver weight
d a change in the substrate specificity of the enzyme
e an increase in bile flow.

SHORT ANSWER QUESTIONS

Q9. Write short notes on three of the following:

a enzyme-mediated dealkylation
b alcohol dehydrogenase
c glucuronic acid conjugation
d phase 1 and 2 metabolism.

Q10. Write notes on the role of three of the following in drug toxicity:

a ethnic origin
b cytochrome P450 isozymes
c enzyme induction
d acetylator phenotype.

Bibliography

CALDWELL, J. and JAKOBY, W. B. (Eds) (1983) *Biological Basis of Detoxication*, New York: Academic Press. Although almost twenty years old, this is an important collection of basic information.

DEBETHIZY, J. D. and HAYES, J. R. (2001) Metabolism: A Determinant of Toxicity, Chapter 3, in *Principles and Methods of Toxicology*, A. W. Hayes (Ed.), 4th edition, Philadelphia: Taylor & Francis.

GIBSON AND SKETT (1994) *Introduction to Drug Metabolism*, 2nd edition, London: Chapman and

Hall. Comprehensive yet concise text on drug metabolism available.

HAWKINS, D. R. (Ed.) (1988–) *Biotransformations*, vols 1–, London: The Royal Society of Chemistry. This series is really a reference work for those interested in specific examples and particular metabolic pathways.

HODGSON, E. (1994) Chemical and Environmental Factors Affecting Metabolism of Xenobiotics, in *Introduction to Biochemical Toxicology*, E. Hodgson and P. E. Levi (Eds), 2nd edition, Connecticut: Appleton Lange.

JAKOBY, W. B. (Ed.) (1980) *Enzymatic Basis of Detoxication*, New York: Academic Press. Although twenty years old now, this is an important collection of basic information.

JAKOBY, W. B., BEND, J. R. and CALDWELL, J. C. (Eds) (1982) *Metabolic Basis of Detoxication*, New York: Academic Press. Although almost twenty years old, this is an important collection of basic information.

PARKINSON, A. (1996) Biotransformation of xenobiotics, Chapter 6, in *Casarett and Doull's Toxicology, The Basic Science of Poisons*, C. D. Klaassen (Ed.), 5th edition, New York: McGraw-Hill.

PRATT, W. B. and TAYLER, P. (Eds). (1990) *Principles of Drug Action: The Basis of Pharmacology*, 3rd edition, New York: Churchill Livingstone. The pharmacology and kinetics sections are useful with some coverage of toxicology.

RONIS, M. J. J. and CUNNY, H. C. (1994) Physiological (Endogenous) Factors Affecting the Metabolism of Xenobiotics, in *Introduction to Biochemical Toxicology*, E. Hodgson and P. E. Levi (Eds), 2nd edition, Connecticut: Appleton Lange.

TIMBRELL, J. A. (2000) *Principles of Biochemical Toxicology*, 3rd edition, London: Taylor & Francis Ltd.

WILLIAMS, R. T. (1959) *Detoxication Mechanisms*, London: Chapman and Hall. Although rather old now, this was the first, classic book on xenobiotic metabolism.

CHAPTER 4

Types of exposure and response

Chapter outline

This chapter will consider exposure of biological systems to chemicals and the pathological consequences of that exposure.

- Acute and chronic exposure. Routes of exposure
- Types of toxic response
  - Direct toxic action – the liver as a target organ; mechanisms of toxicity
  - biochemical lesions
  - pharmacological and physiological effects
  - immunotoxicity
  - teratogenicity
  - genetic toxicity
  - carcinogenicity
- Biomarkers

Types of exposure

There are two basic exposure conditions for toxic compounds: **acute** and **chronic** exposure. Acute exposure applies to a single episode where a particular amount of a substance such as with an overdose of a drug, enters the organism. Chronic exposure applies to repeated exposure to a substance which may then accumulate or cause a cumulative toxic effect.

Acute toxicity usually applies to a toxic event which occurs soon after acute or limited exposure; chronic toxicity may apply to an event which occurs many weeks, months or years after exposure to either repeated doses or possibly after an acute exposure to a particular toxic substance.

Route of exposure

Routes of exposure have already been discussed in Chapter 2 and so only brief mention will be made here. Exposure via the **gastrointestinal tract** is the most important route for most drugs, food additives and contaminants, natural products, and other potentially toxic substances. **Inhalation** is particularly important in an industrial environment both inside and outside the factory and pesticides may also be taken in this way during spraying. Absorption via the **skin** is also important in an industrial and agricultural setting.

The site and route of absorption is important from two points of view:

1 the **route** may influence the eventual systemic toxicity as already indicated in Chapter 2;

2 the **site** may be important if there is local toxicity at the point of absorption.

For example, substances which are irritant may cause inflammation at the site of absorption and this may depend on the conditions at this site. Particles such as **asbestos** will cause damage to the cells of the lung by being taken up into them, but will not particularly damage the skin. The skin will tend to be more resistant because of the outer layer of keratinized cells and its poor absorptive properties.

Drugs may also gain access to the body by routes other than those mentioned; in particular, intravenous and intramuscular **injection** are employed in human medicine while intraperitoneal and subcutaneous administration are commonly used in experimental animals. Intravenous and intraperitoneal injection lead to *rapid distribution* to most parts of the body whereas subcutaneous and intramuscular injection usually lead to *slow absorption.*

Types of toxic response

A biological system can respond in many different ways to a toxic compound and death of the cell or whole organism is only one response. Furthermore there may be many different causes of cell death. Although specific examples will be considered in more detail in later chapters, here we will consider the types of response in general. Many toxic responses will have a biochemical basis yet the expression of those responses can be very different. For example, the biochemical interaction between a toxic compound and a nucleic acid may lead to a tumour but in a developing embryo a birth defect could be the result. Alternatively, an interaction with a receptor could cause a major physiological effect such as loss of blood pressure or by inhibiting an enzyme might cause a sufficient biochemical perturbation to lead to tissue damage and necrosis. **Toxic responses** can be divided up into six categories on the basis of the end result:

i **direct toxic action: tissue lesions**

ii **biochemical lesions**

iii **pharmacological or physiological effects**

iv **immunotoxicity**

v **teratogenicity**

vi **genetic toxicity**

vii **carcinogenicity.**

There may be overlap between these types of toxic response and some chemicals may cause more than one type of effect.

For example in many cases biochemical effects will underlie the toxicity and can lead to tissue damage or some other pathological lesion (see paracetamol, Chapter 5 and snake venoms, Chapter 10). However some biochemical effects of drugs or chemicals do not lead to detectable pathological lesions but rather morbidity or death of the organism may occur through biochemical or physiological dysfunction (see salicylate, Chapter 5).

TARGET ORGAN TOXICITY

The **liver** is a common target organ for the effects of toxic compounds (especially direct toxic effects, see below) and serves to illustrate both the reasons that organs are targeted and the mechanisms underlying different types of toxic effect.

The **liver** is a **target** for toxic substances because of:

a its position in the body in relation to its blood supply (Figure 4.1)

b its structure

c its role in intermediary and xenobiotic metabolism

d its function.

Most toxic substances are ingested by mouth and following absorption from the gastrointestinal tract the blood supply is so arranged that the substance is transported straight to the liver via the portal vein (Figure 4.1). Hence the liver is the first organ exposed to the substance (after the gastrointestinal tract itself). The liver receives 25 per cent of the blood from the heart. Once in the liver the chemical will be taken up into the liver cells (hepatocytes) either actively or by passive diffusion depending on the chemical structure.

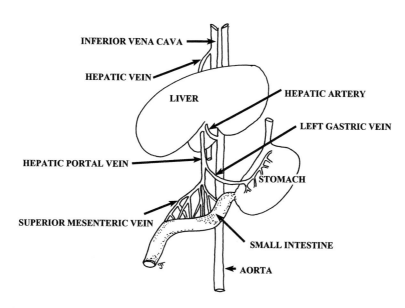

FIGURE 4.1 *The vasculature supplying and draining the liver and its relationship to the systemic circulation. From Timbrell, J. A., Biotransformation of Xenobiotics. From* General and Applied Toxicology, *2nd Edition, edited by Ballantyne, Marrs and Syversen, Stockton Press, USA. Drawing by C. J. Waterfield.*

The **hepatocytes**, which make up the majority of the liver structure, are metabolically very active. They carry out a variety of biochemical reactions essential to the functioning of the whole organism such as protein synthesis, removal of excess nitrogen (ammonia detoxication as urea) and lipid metabolism. Interference with such essential intermediary metabolic activity by exogenous chemicals can result in toxicity. Thus many chemicals that are toxic to the liver inhibit protein synthesis. Two chemicals that cause liver toxicity by interfering with intermediary metabolism are **galactosamine**, which interferes with uridine nucleoside synthesis, and **ethionine**, which blocks the recycling of adenosine in the methionine cycle. Many hepatotoxic chemicals reduce lipid transport out of the liver as a result of inhibition of protein synthesis. For example, the solvent **carbon tetrachloride** causes the accumulation of fat in the liver (**fatty liver** or **steatosis**) via this mechanism.

Hepatocytes are also very active in the metabolism of exogenous (xenobiotic) chemicals and this is another reason why the liver is a target. Many chemicals are metabolized and in the process reactive intermediates may be produced. As these are produced within the liver cell this is the first target. An example of a chemical that is toxic to the liver as a result of this type of mechanism is **carbon tetrachloride** which is metabolized to a reactive free radical that damages the endoplasmic reticulum, and hence disrupts protein synthesis (see above). Other examples are paracetamol (see Chapter 5) and vinyl chloride (see Chapter 6).

The final reason why the liver is a target organ for toxicity is because it also has an excretory function, producing **bile**, which incorporates and transports waste products. Therefore xenobiotics or their metabolites may be excreted by this route. As this is often an active process, the concentration reached in the bile itself may be quite high. This can lead to direct damage to the bile duct. Alternatively, high doses of a chemical normally excreted into the bile may saturate the excretory processes leading to accumulation and high concentrations in the hepatocyte. An example of a compound that causes toxicity by this route is the diuretic drug **furosemide** that causes dose-dependent liver necrosis in animals as a result of **accumulation** in the liver. Other common target organs for the toxic effects of chemicals are the **kidney** and the **lungs**. Like the liver, the kidney also has a relatively high metabolic activity and blood flow and is an excretory organ. Compounds that cause kidney damage are those which are concentrated there such as **cadmium** (see below, Chapter 6) and the drug **gentamycin**. The industrial chemical **hexachlorobutadiene** undergoes further metabolism in the kidney and the reactive metabolite produced damages the mitochondria in proximal tubular cells.

The lungs are targets for chemicals particularly as a result of direct exposure, being the organs of absorption for volatile and particulate substances such as asbestos (see below, Chapter 6). However, they also have a particularly high blood flow and significant metabolic activity. The lungs may be a target as a result of high oxygen concentrations or particular uptake mechanisms such as occurs with paraquat (see below, Chapter 8). In all three organs the cells comprising them are readily exposed to chemicals and able to take up the substances. This is not the case with some organs such as the brain which is organized to exclude many substances, having a 'blood–brain barrier'.

The basic mechanisms underlying toxic responses are similar in all organs and can be divided into primary, secondary and tertiary. **Primary events** are those occurring at the molecular level such as **covalent binding** to crucial macromolecules or **lipid peroxidation**. These may cause enzyme inhibition or depletion of **thiols** (e.g. glutathione) for example.

Secondary events resulting from this are damage to macromolecules such as DNA or changes in the structure or function of organelles such as the mitochondrion or endoplasmic reticulum. These underlie the **tertiary events** such as blebbing, necrosis, apoptosis or steatosis.

Several of the types of toxic response that a tissue can undergo and the mechanisms underlying them can again be illustrated by the liver, with the obvious exception of teratogenesis because this specifically relates to the developing organism (embryo or foetus). Thus, the liver can undergo irreversible destruction of its cells (see Chapter 5, paracetamol), reversible biochemical disturbances such as fatty liver, immune-mediated damage (see Chapter 5, halothane) or develop cancer (see Chapter 6, vinyl chloride).

DIRECT TOXIC ACTION: TISSUE LESIONS

Direct toxicity to tissues, results in tissue damage often manifested as necrosis. This is a process in which the cells are destroyed, the surrounding tissue is often affected and an inflammatory response occurs which can be observed by microscopy. **Necrosis** is an irreversible process during which the cell degenerates, the nucleus may become fragmented and proteins denature. The cells swell, accumulating fluid, lyse and the contents leak out. The underlying mechanism may involve derangement of a biochemical pathway or the production of a reactive intermediate which interacts directly with cellular components such as enzymes or structural proteins or may have an immunological basis. Highly reactive compounds may also react with cell membranes and cause instant cell death by damaging the membrane sufficiently to allow rapid loss of contents and influx of external ions and other substances. Some toxic compounds interfere directly with vital cellular functions such as respiration, which usually leads to rapid cell death. Not all toxic compounds act in this way, however, and some cause cell death to occur more slowly (see lead, Chapter 9). However, the intermediate stages between the interaction of the toxicant or its metabolite with cellular constituents and destruction of the cell are often not clearly understood.

An alternative mode of cell death is **apoptosis**, also known as programmed cell death. This is part of normal tissue turnover and renewal but may also be stimulated by toxic chemicals. One apparent function of apoptosis is to remove damaged DNA which cannot be repaired and this may be one of the triggers that stimulates the process. Severe damage to the cell can compromise the apoptic process and then necrosis may follow. Apoptosis is a process which involves the production of specific proteins resulting from expression of particular genes (e.g. *Fos, myc, max* and *jun.*) The process involves condensation of chromatin and cytoplasmic components. DNA is broken up into small fragments and cell division is blocked. The end result is that the cell contracts away from its neighbours and is removed by phagocytosis. Consequently, there is no inflammatory response.

Skin disease is the most common injury associated with industrial chemicals (see Chapter 6) and most chemical-induced skin reactions are probably associated with direct toxicity leading to irritation. After a single insult to the epidermis the primary response is a local inflammatory reaction. Acute inflammation is the immediate response to irritant chemicals and it is characterized by dilation of blood vessels, increased blood flow, accumulation of fluid in the tissues and invasion of white blood cells. These changes give rise to redness, heat, pain and swelling.

Corrosive chemicals such as sodium hydroxide, cause destruction of tissues (see Chapter 11).

BIOCHEMICAL LESIONS

Biochemical lesions may lead to the development of pathological change such as cell degeneration but they may also simply cause death of the whole organism by interfering with some vital function such as respiration. For example, **cyanide** causes death of cells by interfering with the electron transport chain in the mitochondria such that oxygen cannot be utilized, leading to the death of cells in vital organs such as the heart and brain so that the whole organism dies. Some biochemical effects are reversible, such as the binding of **carbon monoxide** to haemoglobin which may not be at a sufficiently high level to cause death of the organism. Carbon monoxide does not normally cause pathological damage, except at high levels of exposure from which the victim rarely recovers (see carbon monoxide, Chapter 11).

A common toxic response in the liver resulting from a disturbance of normal intermediary metabolism of lipid is **fatty liver** (see above). Other tissues such as the heart and kidney may also show this response to chemical exposure. A more specific type of derangement is **phospholipidosis** in which phospholipids accumulate and which may occur in several tissues, but particularly the lungs and adrenal glands. The drugs **chlorphentermine** and amiodarone may cause this. As well as such pathological changes which can be demonstrable by microscopy, biochemical lesions can cause physiological effects or death by organ failure. For example, **aspirin** overdose leads to biochemical and physiological derangements (ATP depletion, acidosis, hyperthermia) which can lead to death (see below, Chapter 5). **Fluoroacetate**, the natural product which is used as a rodenticide, blocks Krebs' cycle (see below, Chapter 8). This fairly rapidly causes death to animals that have ingested it, probably due to heart failure.

PHARMACOLOGICAL AND PHYSIOLOGICAL EFFECTS

Pharmacological and physiological responses are those where a particular bodily function is affected. For example, some compounds cause a change in blood pressure by affecting β-**adrenoceptors** or by causing vascular dilatation or constriction. These clearly are toxic reactions if extreme and directly life threatening or when they occur in workers occupationally exposed to the drug for example. Alternatively, a drop in blood pressure may be sufficient to initiate another response such as ischaemic tissue damage due to insufficient blood flow. (See **debrisoquine** and **succinyl choline**, Chapter 5 and **tetrodotoxin** and **botulinum toxin**, Chapter 10.)

IMMUNOTOXICITY

Toxic reactions involving the immune system may be manifested in a number of ways: as **hypersensitivity** or **allergic reactions** and **autoimmunity**, which are categorized as indirect immunotoxicity and **immunosuppression** and **immunostimulation** which are categorized as direct immunotoxicity. Hypersensitivity or allergic reactions may occur when the immune system is stimulated after individuals are exposed to chemicals which may bind to or alter a macromolecule, commonly a protein. The protein must be large enough and have sufficient hapten groups attached to be regarded as foreign by the immune system and so act as an **antigen**. Most commonly the chemical (known as a **hapten**) reacts with and becomes attached to an endogenous macromolecule such as a protein which is then regarded as foreign. Allergic reactions may develop at the site of exposure such as the lungs or skin or may cause a systemic reaction. For example, **toluene diisocyanate**, an industrial chemical, will cause allergic type reactions as a result of exposure of the lungs. Immune reactions take one of several forms, including stimulation of a physiological response such as bronchoconstriction, or cellular destruction by complement. The hepatotoxicity of **halothane** and the adverse effects of **hydralazine** are examples of autoimmune reactions where a body constituent is attacked by the immune system (see Chapter 5). An immune-mediated reaction

may underly rare, idiosyncratic, responses (see halothane, Chapter 5) or more common adverse effects of drugs (see hydralazine, Chapter 5). **Penicillin** is the drug most commonly associated with allergic reactions which may take a number of different forms ranging from severe and possibly fatal anaphylactic shock to skin rashes.

There are four different types of hypersensitivity reactions as shown in Figure 4.2, but these will not be discussed in detail. **Type I reactions (anaphylaxis)** may be elicited by chemicals such as **penicillin** and **toluene diisocyanate**. Sensitization occurs after initial exposure and then subsequent exposures cause the anaphylactic reaction resulting in

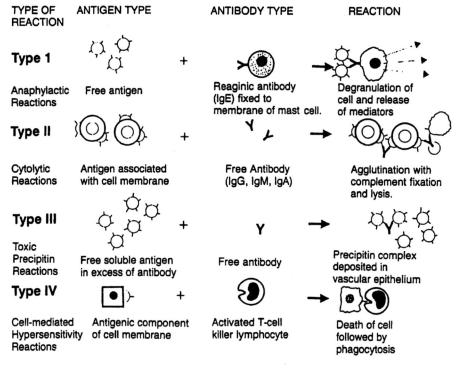

FIGURE 4.2 *Mechanisms for the stimulation of an immune response. The antigen is usually a foreign macromolecule such as a protein or an altered cell membrane as in Type IV reactions. Most foreign compounds are of low molecular weight and are not directly antigenic. They may act as haptens and so cause immune reactions by reacting with and thereby altering endogenous proteins or cell membrane components.*
Adapted from Bowman, W. C. and Rand, M. J., Textbook of Pharmacology, *2nd edition, Blackwells Scientific Publishers, Oxford.*

bronchoconstriction and asthma, for example. **Type II** reactions involve antigens bound to blood cells and so may result in loss of these cells by lysis or removal, such as may occur after administration of the drug **aminopyrine**. A **Type III** reaction may be responsible for the adverse effects of **hydralazine** (see below, Chapter 5). **Type IV** reactions may underlie contact dermatitis, which is a major industrial problem associated with exposure to **nickel** and **cadmium**.

Immunosuppression is the result of a direct effect on the immune system so that it does not function properly. This may be the result of damage to a component of the system such as the thymus, which produces B lymphocytes, or the bone marrow, which is responsible for the production of blood cells. The industrial and environmental contaminant **dioxin (TCDD)** is a powerful immunosuppressant causing damage to the thymus and hence reducing the production of lymphocytes.

Immunostimulation is where the immune system responds to an administered protein, which, although it may be similar to that found in a human, is recognized as an antigen. **Novel peptide drugs** such as those derived from recombinant DNA may elicit this type of immune response.

TERATOGENICITY

Teratogenicity is a very specific type of toxic response whereby the development of the embryo or foetus is affected. This may lead to a functional and/or structural abnormality of the foetus and the resulting animal. Although cytotoxic compounds may be teratogenic, in many cases the malformations are the result of a perturbation in the development of the organism rather than direct damage to the embryo or foetus, as this usually results in death and abortion.

Teratogens are often relatively non-toxic to the mother but interfere in some specific way with the development of a particular stage of the embryo. The timing of the exposure or dosing with a teratogen relative to the stages of pregnancy is therefore crucial (Figure 4.3; see thalidomide, Chapter 5).

Thus the embryo and foetus are especially sensitive to chemical exposure. The reason for this is that the sequence of events in embryogenesis and foetal development is easily disturbed. Consequently, the timing of the exposure is crucial. Therefore there are several characteristics of teratogenesis:

1   teratogens are generally **selective** for the developing organism rather than the maternal organism

2   the **susceptibility** of the **embryo** or **foetus** will vary depending on the stage in relation to exposure

3   the abnormalities observed will often be **specific** to the **stages** of exposure rather than the chemical

4   the **dose response** is often **steep** partly because of the mediation of the maternal organism.

In general terms the outcomes of exposure of a developing organism are limited to four:

1   **death** and **abortion**

2   **malformations**

3   **growth retardation**

4   **functional disorders**.

There are many possible mechanisms underlying teratogenesis and a small interference in cellular function may be all that is needed. Occasionally teratogenic effects may develop later in the life of the offspring rather than

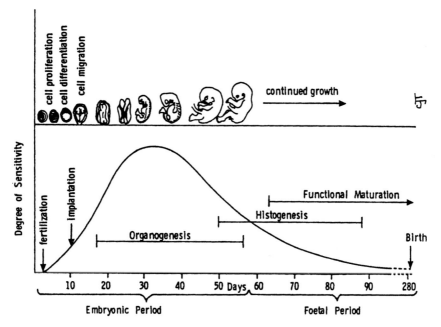

FIGURE 4.3 *The stages of mammalian embryogenesis indicating the periods of greatest susceptibility to teratogens. From Timbrell, J. A.,* Principles of Biochemical Toxicology, *Taylor & Francis, London, 2000.*

during the gestation period. A particularly distressing example of this is the case of **diethylstilboestrol**, a drug once given to pregnant women. The teratogenic effect eventually connected to use of this drug was the development of vaginal cancer in the female offspring of the women exposed to the drug. However, this did not occur until the girls were entering puberty, maybe 12 or more years after their birth and original exposure.

GENETIC TOXICITY

The mutation that may result from an interaction between a chemical and the genetic material is a heritable change in the cell genotype, and thus the error may be transferred to the daughter cell or next generation.

The interactions of chemicals with genetic material can be divided into three types: **aneuploidization**, **clastogenesis** and **mutagenesis**.

Aneuploidy is the loss or acquisition of a complete chromosome; clastogenesis is loss, addition or rearrangement of parts of chromosomes; mutagenesis is the loss, addition or alteration of a small number of base pairs.

Mutations may be characterized as **base-pair transformations** and **base-pair additions** or **deletions**. These refer to small changes in one of the four bases that make up DNA. Thus, in base-pair transformations one base is replaced by another. This may involve replacement of a base by another of the same type (i.e. purine or pyrimidine), in which case it is a base-pair transition. Alternatively, a purine base may be replaced by a pyrimidine, which is a base-pair transversion. This may result in the erroneous coding for an amino acid.

Base-pair deletions or additions involving the loss or addition of a base pair are more serious because the whole base-pair sequence is then altered and the reading of genetic code is shifted. This may result in a **frame shift mutation**.

Large deletions and rearrangements may follow breakage and erroneous reconstitution of the DNA molecule. Similarly, whole segments of the chromosome may become inverted (clastogenesis). These types of changes inevitably lead to major adverse effects in the cell because of the number of genes potentially affected.

Chemicals such as the naturally occurring **vinca alkaloids** may interfere with the process of mitosis or meiosis and, for example, disturb the separation of chromosomes during mitosis (aneuploidization) leading to non-disjunction or unequal partition. This may be the result of interference with spindle formation or some other aspect of the process of cell division. The resulting cell may not be viable, however, leading to cell death and tissue damage.

There are many ways in which a compound may cause a mutation and consequently many different types of foreign compound have been found to be mutagenic. Thus, chemically reactive compounds, such as **alkylating agents**, may *react* directly with the DNA in the cell nucleus, or a compound, such as **bromouracil**, may be *incorporated* into the DNA during cell replication. This may then lead to mistakes occurring in the new DNA. In mammals mutations in the germ cells can lead to birth defects. Mutations in somatic cells are also believed to underlie the development of cancer in most instances (see below).

CARCINOGENICITY

It has been suggested that the majority of human cancers are caused by chemical carcinogens and although this is still a contentious issue, there are now many examples of chemicals which will reproducibly cause cancer in experimental animals.

Carcinogenesis is a specific toxic effect that leads to the uncontrolled proliferation of cells in a tissue or organ. It comes in many different forms, differing in malignancy and type of tissue affected.

Many, but by no means all, chemical-induced cancers are the result of a mutation in a somatic cell. Thus, toxic chemicals may be carcinogenic by interfering with the genetic control of cellular processes via mutation.

Cancer is now believed to be a **multi-stage process**. This in simple terms requires **initiation** followed by **promotion** and then finally **progression**. Exposure to a carcinogen, such as chemically reactive alkylating agents, **vinyl chloride** and **aflatoxins** (see Chapters 6 and 10, respectively) causes an initiating event. This is normally followed by several exposures to a substance which is a promoter. Experimental studies have indicated that the initiating event produces an irreversible change (such as damage to DNA) and must precede the promotion stage. For example, tumours of mouse skin can be caused by application of an initiator such as **benzo(a)pyrene**, a polycyclic hydrocarbon, followed by a **phorbol ester** (promoter). Several exposures to an initiator may result in tumours in the absence of a promoter. The initiation stage typically involves the interaction between DNA and a reactive chemical. The promotion stage involves an alteration in genetic expression and the growth of a clone from the original initiated cell.

During progression the **neoplastic cells** may change phenotype and become a **malignant tumour** involving increased growth and invasion of healthy tissue. However, not all carcinogens are mutagenic, for example **ethionine** and **asbestos** (see Chapter 6). Therefore mechanisms that do not involve a mutagenic event (**epigenetic mechanisms**) must be invoked to explain the cancer caused by such compounds. Furthermore, not all mutagens are carcinogens, although there is a sufficiently good correlation between mutagenicity and carcinogenicity for mutagenicity tests to be regarded as predictive of potential carcinogenicity (see Chapter 12).

Mutagenicity tests are also of use for prediction of germ cell defects and hence damage that is heritable.

One type of chemical carcinogen that is not mutagenic are **peroxisome proliferators**. This type of carcinogen has been extensively studied, especially as a number of drugs and industrial chemicals fall into this category. Compounds such as the drug **clofibrate** and plasticizers such as **phthalate esters** have been found to produce liver tumours in rodents after repeated exposures. Associated with this effect is the phenomenon of proliferation in the number of peroxisomes. The result is not only an increase in the number of peroxisomes, an intracellular organelle, but an increase in a number of the enzymes located in the peroxisome and an increase in liver size due to hyperplasia. However, clofibrate and other compounds are only carcinogenic in rodents. It appears that the phenomenon of peroxisome proliferation requires a cellular receptor and only those species that possess a functional receptor are responsive to these chemicals. Humans, it seems, do not possess a fully functional receptor.

The mechanism underlying the carcinogenicity of peroxisome proliferators involves a combination of increased oxidative stress due to increased production of **hydrogen peroxide** in the peroxisome and increased cell proliferation. As well as the requirement for a functional receptor, peroxisomal proliferators show a clear dose threshold for both the peroxisomal effects and the tumour induction therefore allowing a risk assessment to be made (see below, Chapter 12).

Biomarkers

Determination of the true exposure to a chemical substance, of the response of the organism to that chemical and its potential susceptibility to toxic effects are all crucial parameters in toxicology. Biomarkers are tools that facilitate measurement of these.

There are thus three types of biomarkers: biomarkers of **exposure** of the organism to the toxic substance, biomarkers of **response** of the organism to that exposure and biomarkers of **susceptibility** of the organism to the chemical. Thus, exposure may be crudely determined by measuring the dose but it cannot be assumed that all of the dose is absorbed. Therefore a more precise estimate of exposure is the blood level of the chemical. The level of a chemical in the blood approximates to the concentration in organs, which are perfused by that blood, one of which may be a target for toxicity. However, a metabolite may be responsible for the toxicity and therefore measuring the parent chemical may not be an appropriate biomarker. A more appropriate marker of exposure would be the **metabolite** itself, or if this was a reactive metabolite, a glutathione conjugate or one of its products which reflects the formation of a reactive metabolite could be measured in the urine. Unlike biomarkers of exposure, which are relatively few for a particular chemical, there are many biomarkers of response which may be measured. These include markers such as **enzymes** which appear in the blood when an organ is damaged, increased levels of an enzyme or stress protein (induction), urinary constituents, enzyme activity and pathological changes detected at the gross, microscopic and subcellular level. Indeed, a biomarker of response could be almost any indication of altered structure or function. The search for novel biomarkers now includes study of changes in genes (**genomics**), changes in the proteins produced from them (**proteomics**) and changes in the metabolites resulting from these proteins (**metabonomics**).

Finally, biomarkers of susceptibility can be determined for example in individual members of a population. This could be a **genetic defi-**

ciency in a particular enzyme involved in detoxication or xenobiotic metabolism such as CYP 2D6 or N-acetyltransferase for example. A less common type of susceptibility marker is that reflecting increased responsiveness of a receptor or resulting from a metabolic disorder, such as glucose 6-phosphate dehydrogenase deficiency, leading to increased susceptibility. These three types of biomarkers are all inter-related as indicated in Figure 4.4.

Summary and learning objectives

In this chapter **types of exposure** and **types of response** have been discussed. Exposure to chemicals may be either **acute** or **chronic** as will be the responses. Routes of exposure may affect the type and location of the response which can be local or systemic. Biological systems can respond in many different ways ranging from simple irritation to complex immunological reactions. The major types of toxic responses observed are: direct toxic action; tissue lesions; biochemical lesions; pharmacological or physiological effects; immunotoxicity; teratogenicity; genetic toxicity; carcinogenicity.

Certain organs may be **targets** for toxicity, such as the **liver**. This is due to its position in the body, structure, role in metabolism and function. Hepatocytes are metabolically very active cells and the liver is crucial to the organism. Liver may suffer steatosis, necrosis, damage to the biliary system. Kidney is also often a tar-

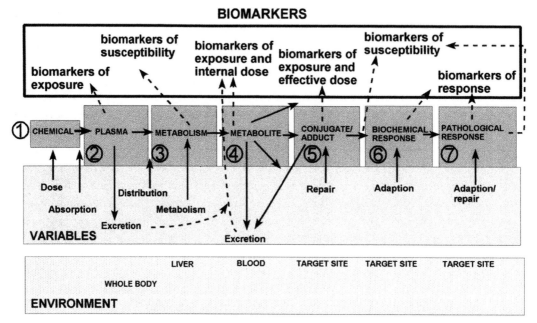

FIGURE 4.4 *The three types of biomarkers and their interrelationships. The numbers represent stages from initial exposure of the organism (1), through absorption into the plasma (2), metabolism of the chemical (3), distribution and interaction of a metabolite with body constituents (4), possible formation of conjugates and adducts with macromolecules (5), production of a biochemical response (6) leading possibly to a pathological response (7). Biomarkers may be measured at several different points in the sequence.*
From Waterfield, C. J. and Timbrell, J. A., Biomarkers – An overview, General and Applied Toxicology, *2nd Edition, edited by Ballantyne, Marrs and Syversen, Stockton Press, USA.*

get due to its high metabolic activity and role in excretion. Toxic effects in organs and tissues may involve primary (e.g. lipid peroxidation), secondary (e.g. damage to specific proteins or DNA) and tertiary events (e.g. necrosis).

Direct tissue damage and destruction can result from *local corrosion* or *systemic effects* leading to liver necrosis for example (see paracetamol, Chapter 5, snake venoms, Chapter 10). This is often due to direct interaction with macromolecules. Another form of cell death is apoptosis.

Biochemical lesions are due to interference with a specific enzyme or pathway which leads to cell dysfunction and possibly death of the organism (see Chapter 5, aspirin; Chapter 7, fluoroacetate; Chapter 10, cyanide). Some effects are reversible such as the interaction of carbon monoxide with haemoglobin with no apparent effects if not lethal. Pathological lesions such as steatosis and phospholipidosis are the result of biochemical lesions.

Pharmacological or physiological effects such as changes in blood pressure or vascular dilation are often due to overdoses of drugs (see debrisoquine Chapter 5) with specific biological actions. However, effects such as bronchoconstriction and production of excessive amounts of secretions may also occur with other chemicals such as organophosphate pesticides (see Chapter 8).

Immunotoxic effects may involve allergic reactions, autoimmune reactions, immunosuppression or hypersensitivity. Allergic reactions require an antigenic protein. Immune stimulation may be divided into four types, including anaphylaxis and cell-mediated reactions (e.g. hydralazine, halothane). Autoimmune reactions result in destruction of body constituents (see Chapter 5, halothane). Immunosuppression is a direct effect on a component of the immune system such as lymphocytes or bone marrow (e.g. dioxin).

Teratogenesis is the specific interference with the development of the embryo and foetus in the uterus resulting in a structural or functional abnormality. These can be manifested as abortion, malformations, growth retardation or functional disorders (see Chapter 5, thalidomide). Teratogens are selective, specific for the embryo/foetus, often showing steep dose–response relationships. The malformations that result will depend on the stage during exposure.

Genetic toxicity is the specific interference with the genetic material of the cell to cause a heritable change in the cell genotype. There are three types of interaction: aneuploidization (loss or acquisition of complete chromosome), clastogenesis (loss, addition or rearrangement of parts of chromosomes) and mutagenesis (loss, addition or alteration of a small number of base pairs). Aneuploidy and clastogenesis usually lead to major cellular effects. Base pair changes may lead to small changes or consequences such as frame shift mutations. Mutations can lead to tumours.

Carcinogenesis is the production of a malignant tumour, resulting from the uncontrolled proliferation of cells, as a response to chemical exposure (see vinyl chloride, Chapter 6; arsenic, Chapter 9; aflatoxin, Chapter 7) but carcinogens are not necessarily mutagens (epigenetic mechanisms may be involved, e.g. peroxisome proliferators). Carcinogenesis is a *multi-step process* involving initiation, promotion and progression. Initiation in which an irreversible change is produced, such as in DNA, must be followed by promotion in which there is an alteration of gene expression and growth of a clone of cells. During progression there may be a change in phenotype when the cells become a malignant tumour.

Determination of exposure, detection of responses and determination of susceptibility to chemicals involves the use of *biomarkers*. Thus there are biomarkers of *exposure, response* and *susceptibility*. Biomarkers of exposure include metabolites and adducts with proteins indicating internal exposure. Biomarkers of response are many and various and range from increases in serum enzymes to the up or down regulation of genes. Biomarkers of susceptibility are more limited and are individual indicators such as the presence or absence of an enzyme or isozyme.

Questions

Q1. Choose one answer which you think is the most appropriate.
     Which of the following is the *most important* in determining the extent of toxicity of a chemical:

   a   chemical structure
   b   dose
   c   metabolism of the compound
   d   excretion of the compound
   e   metabolic detoxication of the compound.

Q2. Indicate which of the following are true. The liver is a target organ for the toxic effects of chemicals because of:

   a   its highly complex structure
   b   its ability to metabolize chemicals
   c   its blood supply
   d   its excretory function
   e   its low levels of glutathione.

Q3. Choose one answer which you think is the most appropriate.
     The most common toxic response the liver shows after exposure to chemicals is:

   a   cancer
   b   cholestasis
   c   blebbing

   d   necrosis of sinusoidal cells
   e   steatosis.

Q4. There are four general types of toxic effect involving the immune system. Indicate which of the following are included:

   a   anaphylaxis
   b   immunosuppression
   c   skin sensitization
   d   autoimmune reactions
   e   bronchoconstriction.

Q5. Choose one answer which you think is the most appropriate.
     Chemicals which are active during the first week of pregnancy after fertilization of the egg are most likely to cause which effect in the embryo:

   a   death
   b   malformations
   c   functional abnormalities
   d   growth retardation
   e   sterility.

Q6. Match the following:

Aneuploidization	addition or alteration of the number of base pairs
Clastogenesis	loss or acquisition of a complete chromosome
Mutagenesis	loss, addition or rearrangement of parts of chromosomes

Q7. Indicate which of the following are true. Biomarkers are used:

   a   to indicate that exposure has occurred
   b   to detect changes in genes
   c   to measure stress proteins
   d   to measure exposure, response or susceptibility.

SHORT ANSWER QUESTIONS

Q8.   List the types of toxic response which a living system may undergo as a result of exposure to a chemical. Give an example of each type.

Q9.   List the four different types of immune stimulation and give an example for one of them.

Q10. Carcinogenesis is a multi-stage process. Indicate what the stages are and explain each of them.

Bibliography

ALDRIDGE, W. N. (1996) *Mechanisms and Concepts in Toxicology*, London: Taylor & Francis. A somewhat idiosyncratic approach to toxicology with information not readily accessible elsewhere.

ALLISON, M. R. and SARRAF, C. E. (1997) *Understanding Cancer. From Basic Science to Clinical Practice*, Cambridge: Cambridge University Press. A very readable account of the basis of cancer and its manifestations.

Casarett and Doull's Toxicology, The Basic Science of Poisons, C. D. Klaassen (Ed.), 5th edition, 1996, New York: McGraw-Hill. Various chapters.

DESCOTES, J. (1999) *Introduction to Immunotoxicology*, London: Taylor & Francis Ltd. A concise introduction to the subject.

DI CAPRIO, A. P. (1999) Biomarkers of exposure and susceptibility, Chapter 86 in *General and Applied Toxicology*, Ballantyne, B., Marrs, T. and Syversen, T. L. M. (Eds), 2nd edition, Basingstoke: Macmillan.

General and Applied Toxicology, edited by Ballantyne, B., Marrs, T. and Syversen, T. L. M., 2nd edition, Basingstoke: Macmillan. Various chapters.

GLAISTER, J. R. (1986) *Principles of Toxicological Pathology*, London: Taylor & Francis. Comprehensive coverage of pathology from a toxicology point of view.

GREALLY, J. F. and SILVANO, V. (Eds) (1983) *Allergy and Hypersensitivity to Chemicals*. WHO, Copenhagen; CEC, Luxembourg.

HODGSON, E. and LEVI, P. E. (Eds) (1994) *Introduction to Biochemical Toxicology*, 2nd edition, Norwalk, Connecticut: Appleton and Lange.

HODGSON, E., BEND, J. and PHILPOT, R. M. (Eds) (1979–) *Reviews in Biochemical Toxicology*, New York: Elsevier/North Holland. Detailed information about specific toxicants.

PRATT, W. B. and TAYLOR, P. (Eds) (1990) *Principles of Drug Action: The Basis of Pharmacology*, 3rd edition, New York: Churchill Livingston.

Target Organ Toxicology Series, Raven Press/Taylor and Francis. Various monographs.

TIMBRELL, J. A. (1998) Biomarkers in toxicology. *Toxicology* **129**; 1–12.

TIMBRELL, J. A. (2000) *Principles of Biochemical Toxicology*, 3rd edition, London: Taylor & Francis Ltd. Various chapters.

TURTON, J. A. and HOOSON, J. (Eds) (1998) *Target Organ Pathology*, London: Taylor & Francis. One of the very few pathology texts orientated toward toxicology.

WATERFIELD, C. J. (1999) Biomarkers of Response, Chapter 85, in *General and Applied Toxicology*, Ballantyne, B., Marrs, T. and Syversen, T. L. M. (Eds), 2nd edition, Basingstoke: Macmillan.

CHAPTER 5

Drugs as toxic substances

'There are no safe drugs, only safe ways of using them.'
'Doctors put drugs of which they know little, into our bodies of which they
know less, to cure diseases of which they know nothing at all'.
Voltaire

Chapter outline

This chapter will use examples to illustrate the types of drug toxicity:

- Types of drug toxicity
- Paracetamol
- Aspirin
- Hydralazine
- Halothane
- Debrisoquine
- Thalidomide
- Drug interactions
- Altered responsiveness – glucose 6 phosphate dehydrogenase deficiency

Introduction

Most human beings and indeed many other animals are exposed to drugs sooner or later in their lives. However, drugs are substances *designed* to have biological activity and although the layman expects them to be perfectly safe it is not surprising that toxic effects do sometimes occur especially when drugs are wrongly used. However, drugs have made and will continue to make a major contribution to human health and we must accept a measure of risk attached to these benefits.

The tragedy which first made the public and probably also the medical profession fully aware of this unpleasant fact was that caused by the drug **thalidomide**. This event, perhaps more than any other, proved to be a major watershed for awareness of drug toxicity and the need for better legislation and testing of pharmaceuticals. Consequently, we will consider this as one of our examples which will also serve to illustrate the problem of teratogenesis.

There are several different types of drug toxicity: **adverse effects** or **side effects** occurring during proper therapeutic usage; acute toxicity due to **overdosage**; **idiosyncratic reactions** which occur during proper therapeutic usage but rarely; **interactions** with other drugs or other substances being taken concurrently which lead to toxic effects; and **habitual abuse** of drugs leading to chronic toxicity. Drug overdoses come within the bounds of clinical toxicology as does accidental ingestion of hazardous substances whereas abuse of drugs including their use for murder is the domain of the forensic toxicologist.

The basic mechanisms underlying these types of toxicity may also be summarized:

1 direct and **predictable** toxic effects due to altered or inhibited metabolism and occurring after **overdoses**;

2 toxic effects occurring after repeated **therapeutic doses** with a metabolic, pharmacological or maybe immunological basis;

3 direct but **unpredictable toxic effects** occurring after single therapeutic doses and due to idiosyncratic metabolism or a pharmacodynamic response;

4 toxic effects due to **another drug or substance** interfering with the disposition or pharmacological response of the drug in question.

Examples of some of these types of drug toxicity will be considered in this chapter.

Paracetamol

Overdosage with drugs is now one of the commonest means of committing suicide and one of the drugs most commonly involved in the UK is paracetamol with at least 200 deaths a year being due to overdoses of this drug. As well as intentional, *suicidal* overdoses, *accidental* poisoning has also occurred and recently been highlighted. This occurred as a result of patients and doctors being unaware that some proprietary preparations contain paracetamol. Thus, repeated **self medication** with paracetamol tablets possibly along with cold cures which may also contain the drug has lead to fatal overdosage in at least one case (see *Pharmaceutical Journal,* Bibliography). Paracetamol is a minor **analgesic** which is very safe provided only the normal therapeutic dose of one or two tablets (500 mg) is taken. However, after overdoses, where fifteen or twenty tablets may be taken, **fatal liver damage** can result. Fortunately an understanding of the mechanism underlying paracetamol toxicity has led to a method of *antidotal treatment* which is now able to prevent the fatal outcome in many cases.

Paracetamol is metabolized mainly by **conjugation** with sulphate and glucuronic acid. Only a minor proportion is metabolized by **oxidation** which is catalyzed by the microsomal mono-oxygenases (Figure 5.1). This produces a metabolite which is toxic but is normally detoxified by reaction with **glutathione** (see Chapter 3). However, research in experimental animals has shown that after an overdose several changes take place in this metabolic scheme. The pathways of conjugation are saturated and cofactors, especially sulphate, are depleted. As a result *more* paracetamol is metabolized by the oxidative pathway giving rise to the toxic metabolite. Sufficient of this metabolite is produced in the liver to deplete all the glutathione available. Therefore, the toxic metabo-

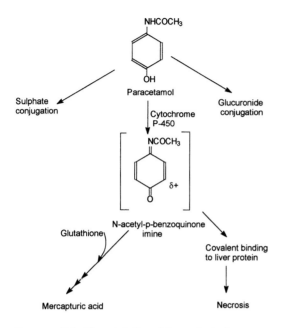

NHCOCH₃

OH
Paracetamol

Sulphate
conjugation

Glucuronide
conjugation

Cytochrome
P-450

NCOCH₃

δ+

O

Glutathione

N-acetyl-p-benzoquinone
imine

Covalent binding
to liver protein

Mercapturic acid

Necrosis

FIGURE 5.1 *The metabolism of the analgesic drug*
paracetamol.
From Timbrell, J. A., Principles of Biochemical
Toxicology, *Taylor & Francis, London, 2000.*

lite reacts with liver proteins instead of the glutathione and this causes direct tissue damage leading to **hepatic necrosis**.

Another factor of importance in relation to the susceptibility to toxicity is individual variation in metabolism, possibly as a result of the intake of other drugs. For example, excessive **alcohol** intake prior to paracetamol overdose may *increase* the liver damage as a result of induction of the particular isoenzyme of **cytochrome P450** involved in the metabolic activation of paracetamol. The elucidation of this mechanism suggested a means of treatment with an **antidote** to either regenerate glutathione or replace it with an alternative. The currently accepted treatment uses **N-acetylcysteine** given either orally or intravenously. Provided this is given within 10–12 hours of the overdose fatal liver damage is usually avoided.

A number of other drugs are taken in overdose for purposes of suicide and these cause various toxic effects. Such drugs include **aspirin, tranquillizers, barbiturates** and **opiates** but antidotes are not available for most of these. Supportive measures, decreasing absorption, increasing elimination or altering the distribution of the drug are the major types of treatment.

Aspirin (salicylate)

Acetylsalicylic acid, commonly known as aspirin, is still one of the most widely used minor analgesics and other salicylates also are used therapeutically. This drug is still an important cause of human poisoning resulting both from overdoses and from therapeutic use. These result in a significant number of deaths each year in the UK and other countries. In children the majority of deaths are from therapeutic overdose. The toxic effects are very much biochemical and physiological, with no clear target organ. However, aspirin poisoning illustrates how chemicals can cause toxicity or even lethality without damaging a particular tissue or organ specifically.

When used repeatedly, aspirin at therapeutic doses may accumulate in the patient and eventually reach concentrations that are toxic. The reason for this is that parts of the metabolism and hence elimination of aspirin are **saturable**. The majority of a dose of aspirin (acetylsalicylic acid) is hydrolysed by esterases to salicylic acid (Figure 5.2). Salicylic acid is then metabolized by conjugation with glucuronic acid or glycine. However, these conjugation steps are saturable and therefore elimination is reduced as the dose increases (Table 5.1). As can be seen from the table, the half-life of aspirin increases significantly even with only a small increase in the number of tablets. This means that a knowledge of the

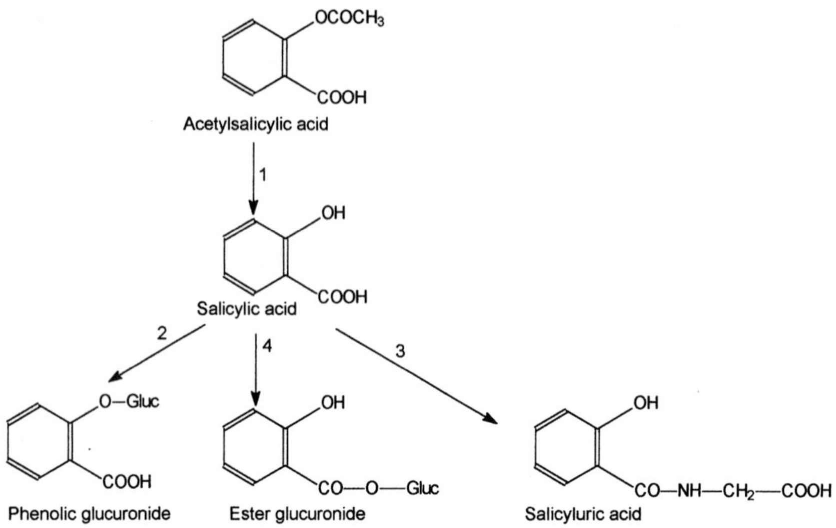

FIGURE 5.2　*The metabolism of aspirin. Step 1 (hydrolysis) yields the major metabolite salicylic acid which is conjugated with glucuronic acid (2 and 4) or glycine (3). Pathways 2, 3, and 4 are saturable.*
From Timbrell, J. A., Principles of Biochemical Toxicology, *Taylor & Francis, 2000.*

blood level of salicylate is very important for the clinical toxicologist.

The primary toxic effect of salicylate is that it interferes with the function of the electron transport chain in the mitochondria, leading to **uncoupling of ATP** production. This leads to a decrease in the production of ATP, increased utilization of oxygen and increased production of carbon dioxide.

This causes the patient to hyperventilate and salicylate also directly influences the control of breathing. These effects result in an increase in

TABLE 5.1　*The effect of dose on the disposition of aspirin and its toxicity*

No. of tablets (dose)	$T\frac{1}{2}$ (h)	V_D L kg^{-1}	Blood level (μg ml^{-1})	Symptoms of toxicity
1 (300 mg)	3	0.1	43	None
2 (600 mg)	4	0.15	57	None
3 (900 mg)	5	0.17	76	None
12 (3.6 g)	6	0.2	25	Tinnitus
30 (9 g)	20	0.25	51.4	Hyperventilation, respiratory alkalosis, metabolic acidosis, fever
70 (21 g)	>20	0.30	1000	Coma, convulsions, respiratory failure, renal failure
100 (30 g)	>20	0.33	1299	Death

$T\frac{1}{2}$: plasma half-life. V_D: volume of distribution.
Data from M. J. Ellenhorn and D. G. Barceloux, *Medical Toxicology*, 1988, Elsevier Science Publishing.

the pH of the blood known as **respiratory alkalosis**. The body corrects this by eliminating sodium bicarbonate into the urine and the pH drops. However, in children and after severe overdoses in adults, the pH may fall too extensively and the patient enters **metabolic acidosis**. This results in a change in the distribution of the salicylate. As salicylate, the main metabolite of aspirin, is an acid, elimination into the urine is sensitive to pH and when this falls, excretion will decrease as reabsorption in the kidney increases. Furthermore, distribution into the tissues, and particularly the brain, will increase as a greater proportion of the salicylate is in the unionized form. This will increase the effect of the salicylate on mitochondrial respiration in tissues and particularly the brain. Overall the patient suffers lack of ATP in crucial organs such as brain and heart, the temperature rises because the energy not used in the production of ATP is dissipated as heat. The excretion of bicarbonate that occurs in response to the rise in blood pH results in loss of sodium and water and the rise in temperature causes sweating.

Consequently, the patient becomes dehydrated. As the urine pH has decreased, the salicylate and its metabolites are not readily excreted and the drug is not eliminated, which worsens the situation. Salicylate also has other effects such as inhibition of parts of Krebs' cycle and increased glycolysis (to produce the missing ATP) which causes further acidosis.

The toxicity is therefore due to the biochemical effects of low levels of ATP and acidosis. Treatment is relatively straightforward and involves reducing the acidosis by increasing the blood pH, giving a source of energy (glucose) and increasing the elimination of salicylate. These are all achieved by infusing **bicarbonate** solution containing glucose. The bicarbonate increases the pH of the blood, causing salicylate to dissociate and diffuse out of tissues such as the brain. It also increases the pH of the urine and this facilitates the excretion of salicylate into the urine and therefore elimination from the body. (See Figure 5.3.) This occurs because the pH of the urine becomes more alkaline and therefore the salicylate in

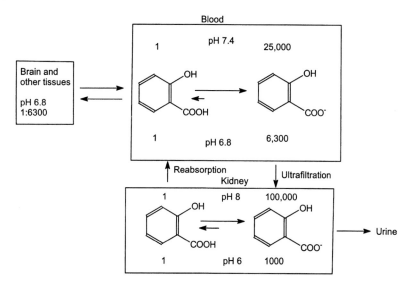

FIGURE 5.3 *The effect of pH on the dissociation, distribution and excretion of salicylic acid. The numbers represent the proportions of ionized and non-ionized salicylic acid.*
From Timbrell, J. A., Principles of Biochemical Toxicology, *Taylor & Francis, 2000.*

the ultrafiltrate produced by the kidney is more highly ionized. Consequently, less is reabsorbed back into the bloodstream. Knowing the pK_a of salicylic acid it is possible to calculate that if the urine pH is shifted from 6 to 8 there is a one hundred fold increase in the ionization of the acid. This is calculated as follows:

Using the **Henderson Hasselbach** equation (see Chapter 2, page 22).

$$pH = pK_a + Log\frac{[salicylic\ acid^-]}{[salicylic\ acid]}$$

The pK_a of salicylic acid is 3; therefore at pH 6 the ratio of ionized to non-ionized salicylic acid is:

$$6 = 3 + Log\frac{[salicylic\ acid^-]}{[salicylic\ acid]}$$

$$Therefore\ \frac{[salicylic\ acid^-]}{[salicylic\ acid]} = anti\text{-}log\ 6-3$$

anti-log $3 = 1000$. Therefore there is $1000\times$ more ionized salicylic acid than non-ionized at pH 6.

At pH 8 therefore the same calculation yields 100 000. It is clear that the salicylic acid is much more highly ionized in the urine at pH 8 than at pH 6 and therefore excretion and elimination from the body is enhanced.

Similarly in the blood at a pH of 7.4 the ratio of ionized to non-ionized salicylic acid is about 25 000 whereas at pH 6.8 it is 6300. Therefore when the patient is suffering from metabolic acidosis with a blood pH of maybe 6.8, there is more non-ionized salicylic acid able to diffuse into the tissues than at the normal blood pH 7.4 (see Figure 5.3).

The technique of changing the pH of the urine and blood in order to facilitate elimination of a chemical is also used to treat other cases of poisoning such as from barbiturates.

Hydralazine

The second example is of a drug toxicity which follows *normal therapeutic dosage* leading to adverse effects in a significant number of patients. This example is of particular interest because it illustrates the importance of the combination of several **factors** in the development of and susceptibility to an adverse drug effect.

The drug in question is the antihypertensive drug hydralazine. This drug causes a syndrome known as **lupus erythematosus** which has some similarities with rheumatoid arthritis. When the drug was first introduced in the 1950s, relatively high doses were used and the incidence of the adverse effect was high, occurring in over 10 per cent of patients. The use of the drug declined. However, use of lower doses in combination therapy reduced the incidence of the adverse effect although a recent report estimates that the true incidence is still unacceptably high with an overall value of 6.7 per cent. Recent studies have revealed that there are several factors which predispose patients to this particular adverse effect.

The factors so far defined are:

1   dose

2   acetylator phenotype

3   HLA type

4   sex

5   duration of therapy.

We will examine each in turn.

DOSE

This has already been mentioned. The incidence of the adverse effect seemed to be more common when doses of around 800 mg daily were used compared with doses of less than 200 mg daily, which are more commonly used now. One recent study showed more clearly that the *incidence* was *dose related*; as no cases were reported at doses of 50 mg daily, there was a 5.4 per cent incidence after 100 mg daily and a 10.4 per cent incidence with 200 mg daily.

ACETYLATOR PHENOTYPE

Hydralazine is metabolized by the **acetylation route** which is a phase 2 metabolic transformation for foreign compounds which have an amine, sulphonamide or hydrazine group (see Chapter 3). This acetylation reaction is under *genetic control* in man and human populations can be divided into individuals of the rapid or slow **acetylator phenotype**. With hydralazine the adverse effect occurs almost exclusively in slow acetylators. As hydralazine undergoes acetylation it is probable that these differences in metabolism of the drug are responsible for the development of the syndrome. It may be that there is more of the parent drug available in slow acetylators which may initiate an immunological reaction. Alternatively, another path-

way of metabolism may become more important in the slow acetylators (Figure 5.4). There is some evidence for this with the oxidative pathway, catalyzed by the **mono-oxygenases** being the most likely route. However there is now evidence that other enzymes, notably **peroxidases** such as those found in leucocytes are also able to activate hydralazine to yield the same metabolites (phthalazine and phthalazinone). However, which, if any, metabolite is responsible for the adverse effect is currently unknown.

HLA TYPE

It was found that the patients who suffered the syndrome were more likely to have the HLA type (tissue type) DR4 than those not affected. That is, the incidence of **HLA DR4** is 60 per cent in those patients with hydralazine-induced lupus compared to an incidence of DR4 in the normal population of 27 per cent. The role, if any of the HLA type in the development of the syndrome is currently unknown; it may simply be a marker which has an association with a gene involved in the predisposition for the disease.

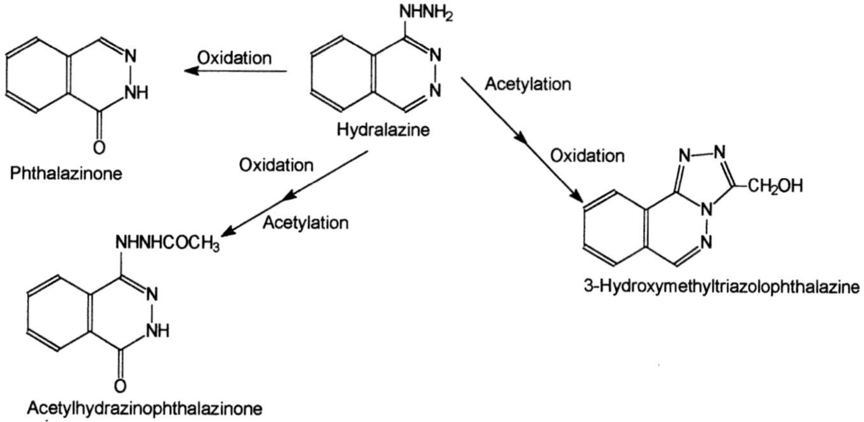

FIGURE 5.4 *The metabolism of the antihypertensive drug hydralazine.*
From Timbrell, J. A., Principles of Biochemical Toxicology, *Taylor & Francis, London, 2000.*

SEX

The adverse effect occurs *more commonly in women* than in men with a sex ratio of about 2:1 overall. However, one recent report quoted an incidence of 19.4 per cent in women taking 200 mg daily compared with an incidence in men of 4.9 per cent when measured three years after starting therapy. Currently there is no explanation for this sex difference as there is no evidence for any difference in acetylator phenotype or HLA type distribution between males and females nor for any difference in metabolism between males and females.

DURATION OF TREATMENT

The final factor is the duration of treatment with the drug; it seems to require an average of **18 months'** treatment for the development of the syndrome.

In view of these factors, the hydralazine-induced lupus syndrome is a particularly interesting example of an adverse drug reaction. The recognition of the predisposing factors allows an estimation of the likely incidence: the HLA type DR4 occurs in around 27 per cent of the population; females account for approximately 50 per cent; slow acetylators are approximately 50 per cent of the British population. Given a sufficiently high dose and duration of treatment these factors give an expected incidence of at least 7 per cent of the normal population. Although true incidence figures are hard to come by, the overall incidence in males and females as recently published is about 10 per cent. Alternatively, it can be regarded thus: a female, slow acetylator with the HLA type DR4 is *very likely to suffer the adverse effect* if a sufficient dose of the drug is given. This means that the adverse effect could be easily avoided if the

prospective patients were screened for HLA type and acetylator phenotype.

The mechanism of hydralazine toxicity is currently unknown although it clearly has features characteristic of an allergic type of reaction. In fact, the adverse effect is usually manifested as a **Type III immune reaction** (see above, Figure 4.2).

Halothane

An example of an adverse drug effect which is a **very rare**, **idiosyncratic**, **reaction** is afforded by the widely used anaesthetic halothane. This may cause serious **liver damage** in between 1 in 10 000 and 1 in 100 000 patients. A mild liver dysfunction is more commonly seen but this probably involves a different mechanism.

The predisposing factors so far recognized in halothane hepatotoxicity are:

1 **multiple exposures**, which seem to sensitize the patient to future exposures;

2 sex, **females** being **more commonly affected** than males in the ratio 1.8:1;

3 **obesity**, 68 per cent of patients in one study were obese;

4 **allergy**, a previous history of allergy was found in one third of patients.

There is now good evidence that halothane causes hepatic damage via an **immunological mechanism**. The antibodies bind to the *altered* liver cell membrane and then **killer lymphocytes** attach to the **antibodies**. In response to this the killer lymphocytes lyze and *destroy* the liver cells of the patient, so causing hepatitis (Figure 5.5). The reactive metabolite involved in the immunological reaction is believed to be **trifluoroacetylchloride** which acylates proteins. This takes place

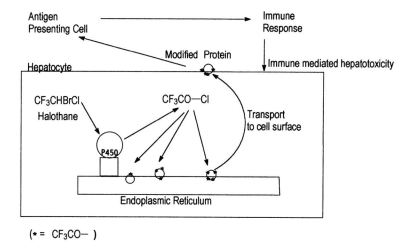

(∗ = CF₃CO−)

FIGURE 5.5 *The hypothetical mechanism of hepatotoxicity of the anaesthetic drug halothane. Halothane is metabolized by cytochrome P450 (P450) to a reactive metabolite (CF₃COCl) the trifluoroacetyl part of which binds covalently to proteins in the endoplasmic reticulum (∗). The metabolite-protein conjugates are antigenic and elicit immune responses in susceptible patients.*
Adapted from Kenna, J. G. and Van Pelt, F. N. A. M. (1994) Anaesth. Pharmacol. Rev. *2, 29.*

in the vicinity of the endoplasmic reticulum and consequently enzymes such as cytochrome P450 are believed to be acylated and become antigenic. Such antigens have been identified in liver.

The more common mild liver dysfunction is thought to be due to a direct toxic action of one of the halothane metabolites on the liver. The exact nature of the toxic metabolite is currently unclear although there is some evidence that the metabolite involved in the direct toxicity could either be a product of reductive or oxidative metabolism (Figure 3.10).

As with hydralazine the knowledge of predisposing factors, in this case the extra risks after multiple exposures, should allow a reduction in the incidence of this adverse drug effect.

The examples used so far have involved a direct toxic effect on tissues mediated either directly or via an immunological mechanism and leading to pathological lesions. The next

example illustrates a type of adverse drug reaction in which a pharmacological effect is involved again with a genetic factor.

Debrisoquine

Debrisoquine is a little used **antihypertensive drug** which was found to show marked interindividual variation. After the normal recommended therapeutic dose is given this drug may cause an *exaggerated* pharmacological effect, namely an *excessive* fall in blood pressure in a few individuals who have a particular genetic predisposition. It has been discovered that about 5-10 per cent of the white population of Europe and North America have this **genetic predisposition** and are known as **poor metabolizers** of debrisoquine. This is due to a *defect* in the monooxygenase system which catalyzes the hydroxylation of debrisoquine at the 4 position, the major metabolic reaction (Figure 5.6). Poor metabolizers have almost complete absence of the cytochrome P450 isozyme which catalyzes the hydroxylation of debrisoquine.

As this metabolic reaction is the *major* route for removal of the drug from the body, such patients have *higher* plasma levels of the unchanged drug after a normal therapeutic dose than normal subjects. As debrisoquine itself is responsible for the hypotensive effect the result is an excessive fall in blood pressure (Figure 5.7). This is another example of unexpected toxicity occurring in a small proportion of the patients exposed. In this case, however, the metabolic mechanism seems fairly clear.

A similar example is the genetically determined toxicity of **succinylcholine**. This again results from reduced metabolism in certain individuals due to an **enzyme variant**. Succinylcholine is a **muscle relaxant** which normally is rapidly removed by metabolic hydrolysis and its duration of action is correspondingly short. In individuals with a *defect* in the **cholinesterase** enzyme responsible for the hydrolysis, however, metabolism is slow and consequently relaxation of muscle is *excessive* and *prolonged*.

Thalidomide

Thalidomide became notorious as the drug which caused **limb deformities** in children born to women who had used the drug during pregnancy. The drug is now a well established **human teratogen**. The thalidomide disaster is particularly important as it was the *watershed* for drug safety evaluation because it was perhaps the first *major* example of drug-induced toxicity. Thalidomide is a **sedative drug**, which was sometimes used for the treatment of morning sickness, and which seemed to be relatively non-toxic. However, it eventually became apparent that its use by pregnant women was associated with a very rare and characteristic limb deformity known as **phocomelia** in which the arms and legs of the infant were foreshortened. It became clear that these deformities were associated with the use of thalidomide on **days 24–29 of pregnancy**. The malformations were initially not reproducible in rats or rabbits and had not been detected in the limited toxicity studies carried out by the company manufacturing the drug. The mechanism underlying the effect is still not understood. Thalidomide is an *unstable*

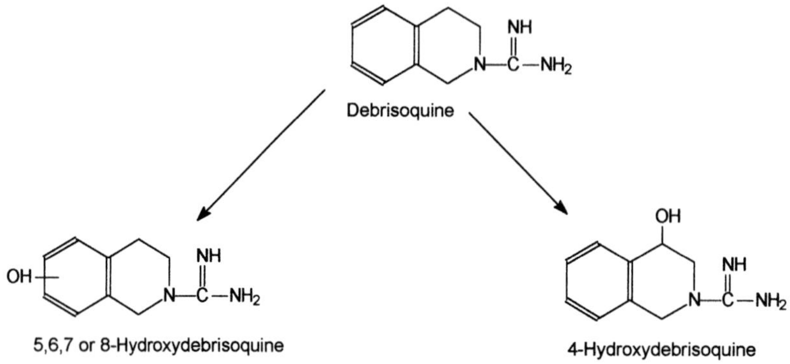

FIGURE 5.6 *The metabolism of the antihypertensive drug debrisoquine.*
From Timbrell, J. A., Principles of Biochemical Toxicology, *Taylor & Francis, London, 2000.*

Debrisoquine

5,6,7 or 8-Hydroxydebrisoquine

4-Hydroxydebrisoquine

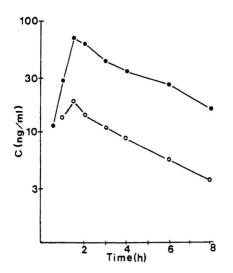

FIGURE 5.7 *The plasma concentration (C) of debrisoquine after a single oral dose (10 mg) in human subjects of the extensive (○) and poor (●) metabolizer phenotypes.*
Data from Sloan et al. *(1983)* British Journal of Clinical Pharmacology, **15**, *443.*

molecule and gives rise to a number of **polar metabolites** which are derivatives of glutamine and glutamic acid but the ultimate toxic metabolite has not yet been identified. Interestingly one of the isomers of thalidomide (the **S-enantiomer**) is more embryotoxic than the other. This is an illustration of the importance of **chirality** as a chemical factor affecting toxicity which has only relatively recently been recognized.

Thalidomide is an exceptionally *potent* teratogen, but because it has very low maternal toxicity in humans and low toxicity to experimental animals it was allowed to be marketed and used as a drug by pregnant women. It was detected as the cause of the deformities from **epidemiological data**, when an astute physician associated the exceedingly unusual effects with use of the drug.

There are many other examples of adverse drug reactions which can be found in the literature and the interested reader should consult the references given in the bibliography at the end of this chapter.

Drug interactions

The problem of interactions between drugs is a major one, particularly with the growth in polypharmacy and **multiple drug prescribing**. Although the physician and the pharmacist should be aware of such interactions new and unexpected interactions can and do appear. Interactions may be due to any one of a number of mechanisms, such as **interference** in the **metabolism** of one drug by another, interference in the **disposition** of one drug by another or alteration of the **pharmacological response** to one drug by another.

Many drugs may interfere with the metabolism of another drug either by **inducing** or **inhibiting** the enzymes involved (see Chapter 2). The best known example is that of barbiturates, such as **phenobarbital**, which induce the mono-oxygenase enzymes and so, by *altering* the *rate* or *route* of metabolism of other drugs, may *alter* their **toxicity**. Paracetamol overdoses are *more severe* if such inducing drugs have been taken, because metabolism via the toxic pathway catalyzed by the microsomal mono-oxygenases is enhanced (see above). Enzyme induction may also *decrease* the pharmacological or toxicological effects of a compound. For example, use of the antitubercular drug **rifampicin**, which is also a microsomal enzyme inducer, increases the metabolism of **contraceptive steroids** and so reduces their efficacy, sometimes resulting in unwanted pregnancies. Whether the toxicity of a particular drug will be increased or decreased will depend on the particular drugs involved and the mechanism of the toxic effect.

Interference in the disposition of one drug by another is a common interaction, particularly involving *displacement* of a drug from a binding site, typically from binding to **plasma proteins**. A well-known example of this is the displacement of the anticoagulant **warfarin** from plasma protein binding sites by **phenylbutazone**, an anti-inflammatory drug. This results in an elevated plasma level of warfarin leading to excessive anticoagulant activity and haemorrhage.

Altered responsiveness: glucose-6-phosphate dehydrogenase deficiency

Occasionally drug toxicity may occur in some individuals due to an unusual sensitivity, i.e. idiosyncrasy. Perhaps the best known example of this is the acute, drug-induced **haemolytic anaemia** due to a *deficiency* in the enzyme glucose-6-phosphate dehydrogenase. This enzyme, which has a major role in intermediary metabolism in the **pentose phosphate pathway**, is important in maintaining the **NADPH** concentration in the red blood cell. NADPH is necessary for maintaining the level of reduced **glutathione** in the red cell, which in turn protects the red cell from oxidizing substances such as the metabolites of certain drugs:

$$GSSG + NADPH + H^+ \rightarrow 2GSH + NADP^+$$

$$\text{Glucose-6-phosphate} + NADP^+ \xrightarrow{G6PD}$$

$$\text{6-phosphogluconate} + NADPH$$

Patients who have this particular genetic defect suffer acute haemolytic anaemia when they take drugs such as the antimalarial **primaquine** or are exposed to certain types of foreign compounds such as **aniline** derivatives. **Fava beans** contain a substance which will precipitate haemolytic anaemia in susceptible individuals, hence the term favism.

The deficiency in glucose-6-phosphate dehydrogenase activity is the result of variants in the enzyme rather than complete absence. The enzyme variants are intrinsic to the red blood cell and so red blood cells from victims will be responsive *in vitro*. On challenge with a suitable drug these red blood cells will lyze and it can be shown that the level of glutathione is *lower* than in non-sufferers and in fact the glutathione level shows a bimodal distribution. It is a **genetic defect** carried on the **X chromosome**, so it is **sex-linked** but the inheritance is not simple. Overall **5–10 per cent** of **Negro males** suffer the deficiency and will suffer acute haemolytic anaemia if challenged with drugs such as primaquine. The highest incidence (53 per cent) is found in male Sephardic Jews from Kurdistan. There are many compounds which will cause haemolytic anaemia in susceptible individuals, some of which require metabolism to reactive metabolites, others not.

Abuse of drugs, alcohol and certain volatile solvents is becoming increasingly common in modern society and consequently so also is toxicity due to this abuse. It is widely known that repeated use of certain drugs leads to habituation and with some drugs to addiction. In some cases the social and related effects of this addiction may be sufficient to indirectly lead to morbidity and death. In other cases actual pathological damage may result as is the case with **cocaine** which causes liver damage and may also destroy the nasal passages when inhaled. The toxic effects of **chronic alcohol abuse** on the liver and brain are widely known as are the many hazards of smoking **tobacco**. Both alcohol and tobacco are addictive drugs and cause far more widespread damage to public health than the more notorious hard drugs such as **heroin** and cocaine. Drug abuse also causes indirect effects on human health, such as injury following driving under the influence of drugs, child abuse occurring as a result of drug use, and the AIDS virus spreading via intravenous drug users.

Summary and learning objectives

Drugs are biologically active molecules to which we are all exposed. They may cause toxicity after **overdoses** (e.g. paracetamol, aspirin) or after **therapeutic doses** (e.g. debrisoquine, hydralazine, halothane). Toxicity after overdoses is often but not always a **predictable exaggerated pharmacological**, **physiological** or **biochemical response**. Toxicity after therapeutic doses is often **unpredictable**, maybe idiosyncratic and unrelated to the pharmacology.

Drug toxicity may be affected by genetic factors that alter disposition or susceptibility and environmental/lifestyle factors such as multidrug use or alcohol intake.

Drug toxicity also may be the result of interactions between two or more drugs or between a drug and another chemical.

Paracetamol causes *liver necrosis* after overdoses as a result of metabolic activation, depletion of glutathione and interaction of a reactive metabolite with cellular proteins. Toxicity may be increased by enzyme induction due to use/abuse of alcohol or barbiturates.

Aspirin toxicity is manifested as physiological and biochemical disturbances (metabolic acidosis, uncoupling of ATP production, rise in temperature, hypoglycaemia). This may follow accidental, suicidal or therapeutic overdosage, the latter resulting from saturation of elimination.

Hydralazine causes an *immunological toxicity* following long-term therapeutic usage par-

ticularly in susceptible individuals (female, slow acetylator phenotype, highest dose, HLA type DR4). This is manifested as a lupus erythematosus-like syndrome with joint pain, skin rashes and antinuclear antibodies.

Halothane also causes an *immunological toxicity* but one that is much more severe than hydralazine. The effect of this autoimmune type of toxic response is destruction of the liver which has a high fatality rate. As with hydralazine there are predisposing factors (female gender, multiple exposures, obesity, history of allergy). The toxicity involves metabolic activation of the halothane, subsequent interaction of the metabolite with liver cell proteins and a combination of antibodies and lymphocytes targeting and destroying liver cells.

The toxicity of **debrisoquine** involves effective overdose as a result of *genetic deficiency* in metabolism. The pharmacologically active parent drug is not metabolized in some individuals (approximately 6–8 per cent of Caucasians) leading to a predictable, exaggerated loss of blood pressure.

Thalidomide caused birth defects (phocomelia) when given to pregnant women for the treatment of morning sickness. It was relatively non-toxic to the women but a potent teratogen when taking during the critical days 24–29 of pregnancy.

Combinations of drugs may lead to unexpected toxic effects as a result of **drug interactions**. These may be due to interference with the metabolism of one drug by another (induction or inhibition), displacement from plasma protein binding sites, or alteration of the pharmacological response.

Drug toxicity may sometimes be due to **altered responsiveness** as is the case with **glucose-6-phosphate dehydrogenase deficient** individuals who suffer haemolytic anaemia as a result of exposure to drugs such as primaquine and some sulphonamides. These susceptible individuals lack the protective glutathione in their red cells, making them prone to damage.

Questions

Q1. Select A if 1, 2 and 3 are correct
Select B if 1 and 3 are correct
Select C if 2 and 4 are correct
Select D if only 4 is correct
Select E if all four are correct

Adverse effects of drugs in humans may be caused by:

1 exaggerated pharmacological effects after overdoses
2 idiosyncratic effects after normal doses
3 toxicity unconnected to the pharmacological effect after inappropriate doses
4 interactions with dietary constituents.

Q2. Choose one answer which you think is the most appropriate.
Paracetamol is an analgesic drug that may cause liver damage after overdoses. This is the result of:

a depletion of body stores of sulphate
b inhibition of cytochrome P450
c production of a glutathione conjugate
d metabolic activation by the microsomal enzymes
e biliary excretion and metabolism by the gut bacteria.

Q3. Choose one answer which you think is the most appropriate.
Which of the following have been shown to be predisposing factors in the toxicity of hydralazine:

a genetic polymorphism of metabolism

b gender
c dose
d alcohol intake
e glucose-6-phosphate dehydrogenase.

Q4. Indicate which are true and which false. Thalidomide is a drug which:

a only causes malformations in rats
b causes morning sickness in women
c causes phocomelia in babies when taken by pregnant women
d is only toxic if the R isomer is taken.

Q5. Indicate which are true and which false. Halothane is a drug which:

a induces cytochrome P450
b destroys lymphocytes
c causes liver damage more commonly in female patients
d causes allergic reactions.

SHORT ANSWER QUESTION

Q6. Why are the plasma and urinary pH crucial in aspirin poisoning?

Bibliography

DAVIES, D. M. (Ed.) (1991) *Textbook of Adverse Drug Reactions,* Oxford: Oxford University Press.
D'ARCY, P. F. (1993) Pharmaceutical Toxicology, in Ballantyne, B., Marrs, T. and Turner, P. (Eds) *General and Applied Toxicology,* Basingstoke, UK: Macmillan.
DUKES, M. N. G. (Ed.) (1977–) *Side Effects of Drugs Annual,* Amsterdam: Excerpta Medica.
DUKES, M. N. G. (Ed.) (1980) *Meylers Side Effects of Drugs,* 9th edition, Amsterdam: Excerpta Medica.
GRIFFIN, J. P: and D'ARCY, P. (1986) *Iatrogenic Diseases,* Oxford: Oxford University Press.

Letter and comment in *Pharmaceutical Journal* (1992) Paracetamol labelling, Kaye, D. F., page 111; Call for more information on OTC medicines, page 114.

STOCKLEY I. H. (1996) *Drug Interactions*, Wallingford: Pharmaceutical Press.

TIMBRELL, J. A. (2000) *Principles of Biochemical Toxicology*, 3rd edition, London: Taylor & Francis Ltd.

WECK, A. L, de and BUNDGAARD, H. (Eds) (1983) *Allergic Reactions to Drugs,* Berlin: Springer Verlag.

CHAPTER 6

Industrial toxicology

Chapter outline

In this chapter you will learn about the hazards of exposure to industrial chemicals using some examples:

- Means of exposure

- Toxic effects

- Vinyl chloride

- Cadmium

- Aromatic amines

- Asbestos

- Legislation

Industrial chemicals

Industrial diseases have existed ever since man began manufacturing on a large scale, and during the industrial revolution occupational diseases became common. Some were well known to the general public and are still known by their original, colloquial names. These diseases were, and some still are of great importance socially, economically and medically. Many occupations carry with them the risk of a particular disease or group of diseases. Thus, mining has always been a hazardous occupation and **miners** suffer **silicosis**, while **asbestos workers** suffer **asbestosis** and **mesothelioma**, and **paper** and **printing workers** are prone to **diseases of the skin**. A man spends on average one-third of his life at work and, therefore, the environment in that workplace can be a major factor in determining his health. Although the working environment has improved immeasurably over the last century, some occupations are still hazardous despite legislation and efforts to improve conditions.

There are now many thousands of chemical substances used in industry ranging from metals and inorganic compounds to complex organic chemicals. The people who work in the industries which use them are therefore at risk of exposure. Fortunately, exposure is often minimized by using chemicals in closed systems so that operators do not come into contact with them, but this is not always the case. In Third World countries, however, some of which are rapidly industrializing, exposure levels are higher and industrial diseases are more common than in the fully developed countries. Consequently exposure to toxic substances in the workplace is still a very real hazard. Furthermore even in the best regulated industrial environment, accidents may happen and can lead to excessive exposure to chemicals.

Means of exposure

Just as with environmental exposure, exposure in the workplace may occur via any or all of the three major routes: by **oral ingestion**, by **inhalation**, and by absorption following **skin contact**. The most common routes of exposure are, however, via inhalation and skin contact. These routes of exposure apply to **gases**, **vapours**, **aerosols**, **volatile solvents** and other liquids as well as to **dusts** and **fibres**. The skin and lungs may come into contact with substances in all of these states and the substances can either be absorbed or cause *local* toxic effects.

Toxic effects

The toxic effects of industrial chemicals may be either **chronic** or **acute**. The acute inhalation of solvents in large quantities can cause **asphyxiation**, **unconsciousness** or **death**, for example. Inhalation of large quantities of very irritant substances, such as **methyl isocyanate** for instance, may cause immediate **bronchoconstriction** and **pulmonary oedema** leading to death. Both of these pulmonary effects are locally mediated rather than systemic effects.

However, such acute effects are usually accidental and so are probably less common than the chronic industrial diseases. They may cause subsequent chronic toxicity, however.

Inhalation of some chemicals, such as industrial gases, metal fumes or organic solvents, leads to irritation or damage to the respiratory tract which may be acute or chronic. In the long term **cancer** or debilitating **respiratory diseases** may result. In the acute phase **irritation** and **allergic responses** may occur. Absorption of substances via the lungs is efficient and rapid and may lead to systemic effects such as **narcosis** from solvents or **kidney damage** from metal salts such as **uranium dioxide**.

Exposure of the skin to some substances in the workplace may cause local irritation, whilst others can lead to **contact dermatitis** or other types of chronic skin disease. Some compounds may be absorbed through the skin and cause toxic effects elsewhere in the body. For example, the insecticide **parathion** has been known to cause fatal poisoning following skin absorption.

As might be expected the respiratory system and skin are the organs most commonly affected by industrial chemicals. Indeed, the most prevalent occupational disease is dermatitis and this accounts for more working days lost in the UK than all other prescribed (see Glossary) industrial diseases together. Dermatitis may have many causes including exposure to organic and inorganic chemicals. Furthermore, chemical agents may act simply as **irritants** or they may be **sensitizers**. In some cases the symptoms may be similar such as the induction of inflammation for example. The number of primary irritants is large and includes many different types of chemical substance such as acids, alkalis, metals and solvents and solid organic and inorganic chemicals. Many of these substances will affect the skin in different ways: solvents will degrease skin, whereas acids and alkalis will denature skin proteins.

Skin sensitizers act via an **immunological** mechanism to cause contact dermatitis. The chemical may pass through the epidermis and react with proteins such as keratin, to produce an antigen. This 'foreign', antigenic protein then initiates the production of antibodies. Re-exposure to the substance will then initiate an allergic reaction. There are a large number of sensitizers of many different chemical types as shown in Table 6.1. **Nickel** and its salts are a well-known cause of contact dermatitis (nickel itch). This may result from occupational exposure and also from exposure to nickel in jewellery.

Sensitization may also be a problem following inhalation exposure where it may lead to a systemic effect such as asthma. **Toluene-diisocyanate** is a **pulmonary sensitizer** which is widely used in industry.

Some compounds such as the **chlorinated hydrocarbons** cause occupational **acne**, which results from plugging of the pores and increased production of keratin.

Vinyl chloride

Vinyl chloride or vinyl chloride monomer (VCM) as it is commonly known is the starting point in the manufacture of the ubiquitous plastic polyvinyl chloride **(pvc)**. This plastic was introduced a number of years ago and there have been many workers exposed or potentially exposed to vinyl chloride during the course of their working lives. However, safety standards in factories and working practices have not always been as rigorous as they are today and were perhaps not always observed. In some cases workers were required to enter reaction vessels periodically to clean them, despite the fact that they still contained substantial traces of vinyl chloride. As vinyl chloride is a gas it can be inhaled but is also readily absorbed through the skin. This was sufficient for some of the workers to be overcome by solvent **narcosis**. The chronic toxic effect of this was not immediately apparent but the most severe lesion, a liver tumour known as **haemangiosarcoma**, was very rare and was observed only in epidemiological studies of workers in this industry. This tumour was generally confined to workers exposed to extremely high concentrations of vinyl chloride. This type of liver tumour has now also been produced in experimental animals. The hygiene and safety standards applied to working with vinyl chloride are now stricter. However, this occurred with the benefit of hindsight and with more foresight the tragedy might have been avoided.

TABLE 6.1 *Types of skin sensitizers*

Type	Chemical class/example
Dye intermediaries	Aniline compounds
Dyes	*p*-Phenylenediamine
Photographic developers	Hydroquinone
Anti-oxidants	o- and *p*-toluidine
Insecticides	Organophosphorus compounds
Resins	Urethane
Coal tar derivatives	Anthracene
Explosives	Picric acid
Metals	Nickel, Chromium

Chronic exposure to vinyl chloride results in 'vinyl chloride disease' which comprises **Raynauds phenomenon** (see Glossary), **skin** changes, changes to the **bones** of the hands, **liver** damage and in some cases haemangiosarcoma. The bone changes are due to **ischaemic damage** following degeneration and occlusion of small blood vessels and capillaries. The liver may become fibrotic. It has been suggested that the vinyl chloride syndrome has an immunological basis, as **immune complexes** are deposited in vascular epithelium and **complement activation** is a feature.

The toxic effects of vinyl chloride may result in part from *metabolic activation*, as it is metabolized by cytochrome P450 to the reactive intermediates, **chloroethylene oxide** or **chloroacetaldehyde**, which *alkylate* DNA and this may thereby lead to cancer (Figure 3.5). The metabolism is *saturable* and the incidence of liver tumours produced in animals reaches a maximum. The tumour incidence therefore correlates with the amount of vinyl chloride metabolized rather than the dose. The reactive intermediate may also react with other macromolecules and cause the tissue damage seen either directly or via an immunological reaction.

The lessons from this example are that safety standards need to be stringent in factories and that animal studies are important in assessing potential toxicity and highlighting the type of toxic effect that might be expected. This should be known before human exposure occurs. As a consequence of this type of industrial problem legislation is now in force in most major Western countries which deals specifically with industrial chemicals. For example, in the UK all chemicals produced in quantities of greater than 1 tonne have to undergo toxicity testing (see Chapter 12), whilst strict occupational hygiene limits, known variously as **Maximum Exposure Limits** (MEL; UK) or **Threshold Limit Values** (TLV; USA) for industrial chemicals are enforced.

Cadmium

Cadmium is a metal which is widely used in industry in alloys, in plating, in batteries and in the pigments used in inks, paints, plastic, rubber and enamel. It is also found **naturally** and may be present in food although it is poorly absorbed from the gut (5–8 per cent). However, up to 40 per cent of an inhaled dose is absorbed and therefore the presence of cadmium in **cigarette smoke** is more significant. It is an extremely toxic substance and the major hazard is from inhalation of cadmium metal or cadmium oxide. Cadmium has many toxic effects, primarily causing **kidney damage**, as a result of chronic exposure, and **testicular damage** after acute exposure, although this does not seem to be a common feature in humans after occupational exposure to the metal. It is also a **carcinogen** in animals causing tumours in the testes as well as at the site of exposure.

Kidney damage may be a delayed effect even after single doses, being due to the accumulation of cadmium in the kidney, as a complex with the protein metallothionein. **Metallothionein** is a low molecular weight protein involved with the transport of metals within the body. Due to its chemical similarity to zinc, cadmium exposure induces the production of this protein and 80–90 per cent of cadmium is bound to it *in vivo*. The cadmium–metallothionein complex is transported to the kidney, filtered through the glomerulus and is reabsorbed by the proximal tubular cells. Within these cells the complex is degraded by proteases to release cadmium which may damage the cells or recombine with more metallothionein.

The testicular damage occurs within a few hours of a single exposure to cadmium and results in necrosis, degeneration and complete loss of spermatozoa. The mechanism involves an effect on the vasculature of the testis. Cadmium reduces blood flow through the testis and **ischaemic necrosis** results from the lack of oxygen and nutrients reaching the tissue. In this case cadmium is probably acting mainly indirectly by affecting a physiological parameter.

The half-life of cadmium in the body is between 7 and 30 years and it is excreted through the kidneys, particularly after they become damaged.

After acute inhalation exposure lung irritation and damage may occur along with other symptoms such as diarrhoea and malaise while chronic inhalation exposure can result in emphysema occurring before kidney damage is observed. Cadmium can also cause disorders of calcium metabolism and the subsequent loss of calcium from the body leads to **osteomalacia** and brittle bones. In Japan this became known as **Itai-Itai ('Ouch-Ouch!') disease** when it occurred in women eating rice contaminated with cadmium.

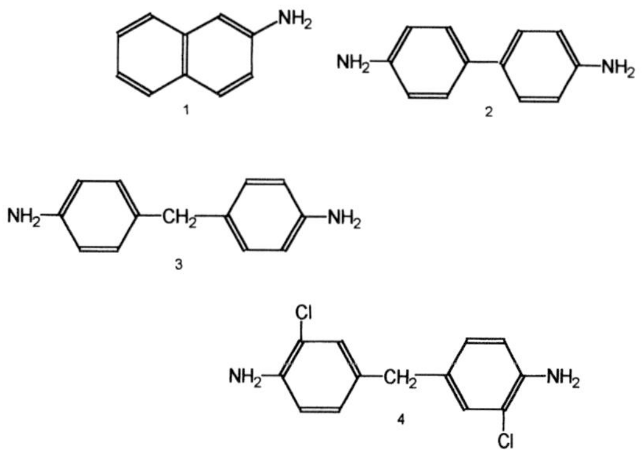

Aromatic amines .

Aromatic amines are widely used in the rubber and dye industry and cause various toxic effects. **2-Naphthylamine**, which was formerly used in the rubber industry is one of the few compounds known to be a **human carcinogen** causing **bladder cancer**. It was withdrawn from industrial use in 1949. The earliest cases of bladder cancer due to aromatic amines were reported in Germany in 1895 amongst aniline dye workers.

There are a number of different aromatic amines used in industry (Figure 6.1) and some of them are known to be carcinogenic at least in animals. However, 2-naphthylamine has been extensively studied and serves as an example. The mechanism of the bladder cancer is believed to involve metabolism. 2-Naphthylamine undergoes hydroxylation at

FIGURE 6.1 *The structures of some carcinogenic aromatic amines. 1: 2-naphthylamine; 2: benzidine; 3: 4,4'-diamino-diphenylmethane (DADPM); 4: 3,3'-dichloro-4,4'-diamino-diphenylmethane, (4,4'-methylene-bis-(2-chloroaniline, MBOCA)).*

the nitrogen atom followed by conjugation of the resulting hydroxyl group with glucuronic acid (Figure 3.15). When the conjugate is excreted into the urine, however, it breaks down under the acidic urinary conditions to yield a **reactive metabolite** which can then react with cellular macromolecules such as DNA.

It has recently been proposed that the **acetylator phenotype** may be a factor in bladder cancer induced by aromatic amines. Acetylation is one route of detoxication for these compounds (Figure 6.2) and consequently slow acetylators would be exposed to more of the aromatic amine than rapid acetylators.

Other aromatic amines used in industry which are carcinogenic in animals are **methylene-*bis-o*-chloroaniline (MBOCA)**, **benzidine**, ***o*-tolidine**, **4-aminobiphenyl** and **diaminodiphenylmethane (DADPM)** (Figure 6.1). This latter compound was responsible for an outbreak of jaundice in the UK, which became known as **Epping Jaundice**. A solution of the chemical was spilt onto the floor of a lorry which subsequently carried sacks of flour. These became contaminated with the substance

FIGURE 6.2 *The acetylation of 2-naphthylamine.*

and people who ate the bread made from this flour became ill with jaundice. DADPM causes bile duct damage and liver tumours in rodents rather than bladder tumours. The target organ for the aromatic amines, however, seems to depend on the species as in rodents liver tumours generally result whereas in the dog bladder tumours occur more often.

Workers who are occupationally exposed to aromatic amines should undergo cytological examination of urine as well as other screening procedures. **Aniline**, the simplest aromatic amine, causes **methaemoglobinaemia** and consequently cyanosis after acute exposure. After chronic exposure anaemia with mild cyanosis may occur.

Asbestos

The industrial diseases associated with exposure to asbestos illustrate that even chemically inert substances can be very toxic. The term asbestos covers a group of fibrous mineral silicates which have differing chemical compositions. It is widely used in industry because of its ability to withstand heat and to provide insulation. **Chrysotile** (white asbestos) is the form most commonly used and is relatively inert biologically but **crocidolite** (blue asbestos) and a common contaminant of white asbestos is especially hazardous as it may cause **mesothelioma**, a rare form of cancer, and also **bronchial carcinoma** (cancer of the lung).

It has been estimated that deaths due to asbestos will peak at between 2–3000 per year in the UK and 10 000 per year in the US over the 30-year period from 1983. There have been more than 400 known deaths from mesothelioma alone in the UK and this cancer is solely associated with exposure to asbestos. Extensive exposure is normally via inhalation in factories manufacturing asbestos products or during its use as an insulating material, such as in power stations and in warships during the Second World War. More recently, workers have been exposed potentially to asbestos during the demolition of buildings in which it has been used. It is widely used in brake linings. The general population is also exposed to asbestos in food and water. It has been used as a material for filters and, hence, may appear in drinks, and it occurs in drinking water in some areas where mining takes place. However, the toxicological importance of this route of exposure is currently uncertain, but gastrointestinal tumours have been ascribed to asbestos after inhalation exposure.

Exposure to asbestos via inhalation can lead to the following conditions:

1 **Asbestosis** or interstitial **fibrosis of the lung**;

2 Benign **pleural disease**;

3 **Bronchial carcinoma**;

4 **Malignant mesothelioma**.

Asbestosis is a dose-related disease and requires heavy exposure for a prolonged period. Particles of asbestos can be detected in the fibrotic areas of the lung and sputum and the air spaces become obliterated with collagen. The asbestos fibres become coated with an iron-containing protein. The disease develops over a variable period of time with breathlessness becoming more severe. Monitoring the lung function of exposed workers in some way, such as by measuring vital capacity, should be carried out as a consistent reduction could indicate the effects of asbestos exposure.

Although asbestos is chemically inert, the fibres are cytotoxic and will haemolyze red blood cells. The length of the fibre seems to be an important factor in the toxicity – **fibres** which are *longer* than **10–20 μm** will cause fibrosis but shorter ones do not. This is due to the *inability* of **macrophages** to *phagocytose* the long fibres fully and so the macrophage cell membrane is damaged and enzymes leak out. These enzymes and other cellular constituents may be involved in the development of **fibrosis**. The lung normally can remove hazardous particles but the long asbestos fibres are not adequately removed and as already indicated they are also not effectively removed by macrophages. An immunological mechanism is also involved and asbestos fibres cause a change in the cell surface of the macrophage after ingestion. This is a change in the receptors for C_3 complement and IgG antibodies. The complement pathway is also activated.

In the UK there is legislation to control the use of asbestos and workers must have a medical examination before and at regular intervals during their exposure. Crocidolite is no longer used in the UK, the use of amosite (brown asbestos) is not encouraged, and the general use of asbestos for insulation will probably be banned. The control limit for crocidolite and amosite in the environment is 0.2 fibres per ml and 0.5 fibres per ml for other forms of asbestos.

Bronchial carcinoma may result from prolonged exposure to asbestos and occurs in approximately 50 per cent of those workers who develop asbestosis. As well as the dose and duration of exposure, the type of exposure is also important. The use of asbestos products, such as in textiles, where asbestos of a particular particle size is generated, is probably important in the development of the disease.

Mesothelioma is a rare form of cancer which affects the chest lining and is associated only with exposure to asbestos, especially but not exclusively, crocidolite. **Crocidolite** from the north-west Cape Province in South Africa is more *potent* than that from the Transvaal. Prolonged exposure to high levels of asbestos is not necessary for the development of mesothelioma and it has developed in people not occupationally exposed to asbestos. Although the latent period is usually long, typically 30 years after exposure, once diagnosed the disease is usually fatal within months rather than years. The tumour may eventually spread to the lung and may eventually encase it.

The mechanisms underlying asbestos-induced cancer are currently unknown but do not seem to involve genotoxic mechanisms. Animal studies as well as human data have shown that asbestos fibres alone will cause cancer of the mesothelium. Unlike other types of chemical carcinogen, asbestos is not metabolized or activated *in vivo* but once present in the tissues it remains there permanently although the fibres do migrate from the airways to the pleural cavity. Consequently, even exposure to high levels for short periods of time may be sufficient to eventually cause mesothelioma.

The **size of the fibres** appears to be a critical factor, with those 0.3 μm in diameter and 5 μm in length being the *most active*. The extent of exposure in terms of the concentration of fibres in inhaled air is also important. Other factors have also been identified. There may be a synergistic effect between smoking and asbestos in the induction of pulmonary carcinogenesis.

Legislation

In the UK, the USA and in most other major Western industrialized nations there is legislation which sets limits on the levels of toxic substances in the workplace. This involves setting exposure levels based on the results of human epidemiological data and on the results of animal toxicity studies. It requires monitoring of the occupational environment for compliance. The experimental evidence of toxic effects usually includes, the determination of a dose–response relationship and no-effect levels in experimental animals. Limited studies, such as exposure to solvents for irritant effects, for skin sensitization may, however, be conducted in human volunteers under carefully controlled conditions after ethical considerations have been made.

The maximum level of exposure for a compound is known as the Maximum Exposure Limit (**MEL**) in the UK or the threshold limit value (**TLV**) in the USA. These are calculated on the basis of exposure over a normal working day usually from a knowledge of the toxicity of the compound in experimental animals (**NOAEL**) with a margin of safety included in the estimate (see Chapters 1 and 12). Such occupational exposure limits are set by the regulatory body, in the case of the UK this is the Health and Safety Executive, and these should not be exceeded. The fact that industrial diseases still occur suggests that some factories do not adhere to these limits or that safety precautions such as the wearing of masks are not taken. Unfortunately with some diseases, such as cancer, the development time is long and therefore diseases may occur many years after the initial, critical exposure when safety standards were not as strict as those today.

This long latency period also means that the detection of industrial diseases is often difficult, as there has to be a sufficient rarity and sufficiently increased frequency of the disease within a particular population for **epidemiologists** to detect it. In the UK however, new legislation requires all new chemical substances not already covered by existing legislation (drugs and pesticides) to undergo **toxicological testing** and consequently exposed people can

be screened for the likely toxic effects. In addition, it allows hazards to be identified so that control measures, such as suitable labelling, can be effected. Despite this, however, new occupational diseases will undoubtedly continue to appear resulting from exposure many years ago. Also, new and unexpected toxic effects may also occur.

Summary and learning objectives

Many of the chemicals used in industry are chemically reactive molecules and are likely to interact with biological systems and cause damage in some cases at the site of exposure.

Exposure is most commonly via skin and lungs. *Toxic effects* on the skin such as irritation, sensitization and contact dermatitis as caused by nickel are the most common occupational diseases and in some cases may have an immune basis. Similarly, allergic lung disease such as asthma may result from exposure to industrial chemicals and some extremely reactive irritant chemicals (e.g. toluene diisocyanate) cause pulmonary sensitization, oedema, bronchoconstriction, and maybe death. Certain industrial chemicals cause cancer which may develop many years after exposure.

High levels of exposure to *vinyl chloride* have occurred in manufacturing plants and resulted in rare liver cancer developing some years later. Apart from this vinyl chloride also caused liver damage and effects on skin and bones. The liver damage and cancer are caused by a reactive metabolite produced by cytochrome P450 which reacts with protein and DNA.

Cadmium is an element widely used in industry in various forms. Its toxic effects include kidney damage following oral or inhalation exposure, brittle bones (Itai-Itai disease) and, after chronic inhalation of cadmium fumes, lung irritation and emphysema. In rodents testicular damage and tumours may occur. Cadmium is bound to metallothionein but release of free cadmium from this complex in the kidney underlies the nephrotoxicity.

A variety of **aromatic amines** are used in industry such as the production of rubber. A number of these are suspect or known carcinogens such as **2-naphthylamine**. Metabolic activation by cytochrome P450, conjugation of the hydroxylated product and release of the reactive metabolite in the urine allows interaction of the metabolite with bladder cell DNA. This is responsible for the carcinogenicity. 2-Naphthylamine can be detoxified by acetylation, therefore the slow acetylator status is a factor and slow acetylators are more at risk from bladder cancer.

Other aromatic amines used in industry are also carcinogenic or toxic in other ways (jaundice, methaemoglobinaemia).

In contrast, **asbestos** is a relatively inert substance but causes lung cancer (mesothelioma, bronchial carcinoma) and asbestosis, a chronic lung disease. The fibres lodge in the lungs, are taken up by phagocytic cells which leak cell contents and damage the surrounding tissue. Fibre size is a crucial factor. Exposure to such chemicals and minerals is now tightly controlled by **legislation** and exposure levels (TLV, MEL) are set.

Questions

Q1. Indicate which is true and which is false. Skin sensitization is an important occupational disease and can be caused by:

a vinyl chloride
b cadmium

c nickel
d asbestos.

Q2. Which of the following industrial chemicals are known human carcinogens?

a cadmium
b vinyl chloride
c 2-naphthylamine
d asbestos.

Q3. In order to calculate the TLV for an industrial chemical which of the following are needed?

a latency period
b half-life
c NOAEL
d daily exposure level.

Q4. The toxicity of asbestos is affected by which of the following?

a fibre size
b form of asbestos
c route of exposure
d dose
e exposure period.

Q5. Which of the following is caused by both cadmium and vinyl chloride?

a testicular damage
b kidney damage
c bone damage
d ischaemia.

SHORT ANSWER QUESTION

Q6. Explain how the acetylation and glucuronic acid conjugation are important in 2-naphthylamine carcinogenicity.

Bibliography

ANDERSON, K. E. and SCOTT, R. M. (1981) *Fundamentals of Industrial Toxicology,* Ann Arbor, Mich.: Ann Arbor Science.

Casarett and Doull's Toxicology, The Basic Science of Poisons, C. D. Klaassen (Ed.), 5th edition, 1996, New York: McGraw-Hill.

General and Applied Toxicology, Ballantyne, B., Marrs, T. and Syversen, T. L. M. (Eds), 2nd edition, 1999, Basingstoke: Macmillan. Various chapters.

HAMILTON, A. and HARDY, H. L. (1983) *Industrial Toxicology,* revised A. J. Finkel, Bristol: J. Wright & Sons.

HUNTER, D. (1978) *Diseases of Occupations,* 6th edition, London: Hodder & Stoughton.

Patty's Industrial Hygiene and Toxicology (1978) vols I–III, 3rd edition, New York: John Wiley.

STACEY, N. (Ed.) (1993) *Occupational Toxicology,* London: Taylor & Francis.

WALDRON, H. A. (1985) *Lecture Notes on Occupational Medicine,* 3rd edition, Oxford: Blackwell.

CHAPTER 7

Food additives and contaminants

Chapter outline

This chapter will discuss the toxicology of food additives and contaminants using specific examples:

- Introductory comments

- Tartrazine

- Saccharin

- Food contaminants

  - Aflatoxin

  - Ginger Jake

  - Spanish Oil Syndrome

Introduction

The food we consume daily contains many different substances, some natural, some added intentionally and some present due to contamination. Substances intentionally added to food, 'food additives', are not as recent an innovation as is often supposed; the use of salt as a preservative and spices to disguise poor food has been common for centuries. However, such treatment of food with additives has only reached the current scale relatively recently, with something of the order of **2500 food additives** currently in use. The use of food additives on such a wide scale is now beginning to be questioned by some toxicologists especially as the long-term effects of the substances in question often are not known. The general public also now questions the use of some of these additives and in response to this food manufacturers have begun to supply certain

TABLE 7.1 *Classes of food additives and examples*

Colouring agents	Tartrazine
Anti-oxidants	Butylated hydroxytoluene
Stabilizers	Vegetable gums
Anti-caking agents	Magnesium carbonate
Flavours	Cinnamaldehyde
Preservatives	Sodium nitrate
Emulsifiers	Polyoxyethylene sorbitan fatty esters
Acids/Alkalis	Citric acid
Buffers	Carbonates
Bleaches	Benzoyl peroxide
Propellants	Nitrous oxide
Sweeteners	Saccharin
Flavour enhancers	Monosodium glutamate

foods which are additive-free or contain only 'natural' colouring agents.

Food additives, grouped according to their use with some examples, are shown in Table 7.1. It can be seen that as well as the colouring agents and preservatives there are other types of additive whose function is less obvious. In Europe, permitted food additives are given a number, the **E number**, which also appears on the packaging of the food.

Food additives have many functions but primarily they allow the consumer to buy food at his convenience and the producer to 'improve' the quality. **Preservatives** clearly serve a public health function in reducing the likelihood of bacterial and fungal infections affecting food. The best known of such bacterial infections is food poisoning from *Salmonella* contamination. Preservatives reduce biological and chemical degradation and so allow food to have a longer shelf life. However, colours and some of the other agents added to food are of less obvious benefit to the consumer and may be more important to the manufacturer. Enhancing the attractiveness of food is the main reason given for their use but many consumers have become

sceptical and have demanded additive-free food or the use of 'natural' additives. Although this may satisfy consumers who believe that **natural substances** are intrinsically safe, natural products can be at *least as toxic* as synthetic ones (see Chapter 10). Each 'natural' food additive needs to be assessed individually. As well as preservatives other additives may also have a useful function, such as artificial **sweeteners** which reduce the sugar intake of people with problems such as obesity or diabetes.

As can be appreciated from Table 7.1, food additives comprise a wide range of chemical types from the simple inorganic compounds used as preservatives to the complex organic molecules used as colouring agents and flavours.

In the past, toxic food additives were inadvertently used, such as **butter yellow (4-dimethylaminoazobenzene)**, a dye used to colour butter, which proved to be a carcinogen capable of causing liver tumours in experimental animals.

Clearly food additives have to be tested for toxicity before they can be used and before humans are exposed to them. These tests usually consist of lifetime exposure of experimental animals to the substance at several concentrations, but with the maximum concentration several times greater than that expected to be consumed by humans. However, such testing may not always be predictive as experimental animals may not show the same type of behavioural or immunological effects as does man and absorption, distribution and metabolism can also be different. Also, the administration of relatively large amounts of a substance to experimental animals may lead to accumulation because of saturation of metabolic or excretory pathways. These kinds of problems were encountered with **saccharin** and clearly make the interpretation of toxicological data difficult. Although the quantities of food additives consumed by humans are very small, their consumption may occur over a *lifetime* and is *chronic* although it may be sporadic rather than continuous. This is difficult to simulate in the laboratory animal.

At the present time there is little reliable data on the toxicity of food additives in man but there is much concern on the part of the public and there have been many anecdotal reports of problems relating to food additives, particularly allergic reactions. The incidence of such **intolerance** to food additives in the population at large is uncertain, most data referring to those patients who have symptoms such as **urticaria**. In such patients up to half may be responsive to food additives but the figures show wide variation. There may also be cross-reactivity between additives and also with naturally occurring food contaminants such as between **salicylates** and **tartrazine** (see below). However certain substances have been removed from the permitted list of additives due to animal data indicating toxicity. One example is that already mentioned, butter yellow. A more recent example is that of the synthetic sweeteners **cyclamate** and **saccharin** (see below), both of which suffered from what was interpreted as adverse animal toxicity data and were banned in the USA.

Tartrazine

One well-known example of a food additive, currently in use, where there are possible problems in man is the food colour tartrazine, also known as **E102** in European countries. This is one of the most widely used colouring agents and also the colour most frequently implicated in intolerance studies especially in pharmaceutical preparations. It is an orange dye used as a colour in drinks such as orange juice but also in a wide variety of other foodstuffs and also in pharmaceutical preparations.

The toxic effects ascribed to tartrazine are the induction of **hyperkinetic** behaviour or purposeless activity in children, and of **urticaria** or skin rashes. **Hyperkinetic** behaviour is difficult to diagnose and distinguish from restlessness which may be due to other factors such as hunger, boredom or inappropriate treatment by adults. The causation of this syndrome by food additives is somewhat controversial as some studies have shown an improvement in behaviour after switching to diets, such as the **Feingold diet**, which are free from artificial colours and flavours, whereas other studies have shown no improvement. One double-blind cross-over study of 15 hyperkinetic children found some improvement when the Feingold additive-free diet was used. On the one hand, a major change in dietary habits might be expected to cause behavioural changes; on the other hand, another double-blind cross-over study using objective laboratory and classroom observation failed to find any effect of the Feingold diet. Yet, another trial on 22 hyperkinetic children found a statistically significant improvement in the mother's ratings of their children's behaviour but not in objective tests. According to Juhlin, the one study carried out to the most rigorous scientific standards where objective, non-involved observers were used showed no effect of diet on behaviour.

Urticaria due to intake of tartrazine, however, is more widely accepted as an adverse effect and has been demonstrated in a number of studies. There is histamine release and the symptoms are the appearance of red weals on the skin and itching. A number of other food colours and other types of food additive may also cause urticaria and there may be cross reactivity between other colours such as **erythrosine** and **Sunset Yellow**. A challenge of patients whose urticaria had improved on a colour-free diet with 0.15 mg of tartrazine resulted in 3 out of 13 developing urticaria within three hours of exposure. **Asthma** may also be a symptom of hypersensitivity to tartrazine: a study showed that 11 per cent of asthmatics reacted to an orange drink containing colouring agents.

Tartrazine sensitivity is also often related to aspirin intolerance. Indeed, between 10 per cent and 40 per cent of aspirin-sensitive patients respond to tartrazine with reactions ranging from severe **asthma** to **urticaria** and mild **rhinitis**. The mechanism underlying tartrazine sensitivity is unknown but does not seem to involve a reagenic antibody or the prostaglandin synthesis system. A range of antigenic substances in the diet are absorbed from the gastrointestinal tract but most individuals become immunologically tolerant via a regulatory system which prevents adverse reactions to food constituents and additives. However, *some* individuals seem predisposed to allergic diseases and do not become immunologically tolerant, hence developing adverse reactions to dietary constituents.

Tartrazine is metabolized by the **gut flora** giving rise to several metabolites (Figure 3.12) and the urine of animals fed tartrazine has recently been shown to be mutagenic.

Although tartrazine is probably the food colour most commonly implicated in reports of adverse reactions, several others may also cause adverse effects including the 'natural' food colour **annatto**. Indeed, in one study 26 per cent of patients with chronic urticaria were shown to be responsive to annatto.

Saccharin

This artificial sweetener, first used in the nineteenth century, has been extensively scrutinized over the years and at one stage was banned from use in the USA. As expected of a food additive, saccharin has low acute toxicity, with an LD_{50} of between 5 and 17.7 g kg^{-1} in experimental animals. It is not metabolized and volunteers taking large amounts for several months suffered no ill effects. Two early long-term studies confirmed its safety. Then two studies showed it to be weakly carcinogenic, but these studies have since been criticized as inappropriate. Increased consumption of saccharin and a report showing another sweetener to be carcinogenic prompted further studies to be carried out. In one, saccharin and **cyclamate** were studied as mixtures with doses up to 2500 mg kg^{-1}. **Bladder tumours** were observed and as a result cyclamate was banned. Still further studies were carried out but proved inconclusive. Finally, a comprehensive study carried out by the Canadian authorities showed that saccharin could produce bladder tumours in rats and saccharin was suspended from use by the Canadian and US authorities in 1977. In the USA it was banned under the **Delaney Clause** of the Food, Drug and Cosmetic Act which prohibits the use of any food additive which has been shown to produce cancer in laboratory animals. There was a public outcry against this banning because saccharin was the only general purpose artificial sweetener approved for use and therefore available to diabetics and those with an obesity problem, as well as to other members of the public wishing to reduce their sugar intake. The result was a moratorium on the ban to allow further evidence to be examined. **Epidemiological studies** mostly showed no increased incidence of bladder tumours but some studies did indicate a slight increase of bladder tumour risk. The absence of detectable metabolism of saccharin after chronic low level dietary exposure and negative mutagenicity data were taken to indicate that saccharin was not a classical electrophilic carcinogen. Therefore, any carcinogenicity was probably due to the unmetabolized parent compound acting by some epigenetic mechanism.

It was found in experimental animals that levels of up to 5 per cent in the diet caused no detectable increase in bladder cancer but levels of 5–7.5 per cent did cause a significant tumour increase. However, pharmacokinetic studies have now shown that the plasma clearance of saccharin is *saturated* at the higher exposure level, giving higher tissue concentrations than would be predicted from a linear extrapolation of data from lower dose studies. Consequently, such high-level exposure in animals may be inappropriate as regards normal human exposure. The saccharin case illustrates the wider social aspects as well as the scientific considerations involved with toxicology. There are value judgements to be made and risk must be balanced against benefit. These issues will be addressed in the final chapter.

Food contaminants

As well as intentional food additives, foodstuffs may also contain contaminants. These might be toxic **bacterial** or **fungal** products, toxic **degradation products** from food constituents, such as pyrolysis products resulting from cooking, or they might be substances inadvertently added to the food. There is now great interest in toxic and especially carcinogenic compounds produced as a result of cooking such as the mutagenic compounds **Trp 1** and **Trp 2**, and carcinogenic **nitroso compounds** produced from dietary amines.

Two examples of naturally occurring but toxic food contaminants are botulinum toxin and aflatoxin. Botulism will only be briefly discussed here as it is covered in more detail in Chapter 10 under natural products.

BOTULISM

Botulism is the syndrome caused by **botulinum toxin** from the bacterium *Clostridium botulinum*. This anaerobic bacterium may contami-

nate tinned or bottled food and the toxin is extremely potent. Heating destroys the toxin. For more detail see chapter 10.

AFLATOXIN

The aflatoxins are a group of related mycotoxins produced by the mould *Aspergillus flavus*. There are four toxins, B_1 and B_2 and G_1 and G_2. The mould grows typically on crops such as grain and peanuts in hot, humid climates such as occur in Sub Saharan West Africa and South East Asia. Contamination can be a serious problem and people living in such areas suffer chronic exposure to aflatoxin. People in importing countries are more likely to suffer from acute exposure. There is epidemiological evidence of an association between intake of aflatoxin B_1 and **liver cancer** in humans. Tainted crops are difficult to sell to countries such as the USA and UK which have strict criteria on levels of mycotoxins. Consequently, the tainted crops may then be sold within the poorer producing country or may find their way to famine victims as part of the relief effort.

Animals fed on meal derived from contaminated feed such as peanuts may develop tumours. The toxins were in fact discovered as a result of the loss of turkeys suffering liver damage after being given mouldy feed. Also, traces of aflatoxin have been detected in **peanut butter**, especially that made from peanuts not treated with chemicals to prevent mould growth and consequently sold in health food shops labelled as '**natural**'.

Aflatoxin B_1 is a very potent liver carcinogen and hepatotoxin; a level of 1 ppb in the diet may be sufficient to cause liver tumours. Levels of aflatoxin in the diet are higher (ppm as opposed to ppb) in Africa than in other parts of the world and this explains the higher incidence of liver cancer in certain parts of Africa.

The mechanism of toxicity of aflatoxin B_1 involves metabolism to a chemically **reactive intermediate** (an **epoxide**) which binds covalently to protein but which also interacts with nucleic acids. This chemically reactive intermediate may be responsible for both the liver necrosis and the liver tumours.

PTAQUILOSIDE

See Chapter 10 for a discussion of this naturally occurring carcinogen found in edible bracken fern shoots.

GINGER JAKE

Then he would eat of some craved food until he was sick; or he would drink Jake or whiskey until he was shaken paralytic with red wet eyes …
John Steinbeck, *The Grapes of Wrath*

Tri-orthocresyl phosphate is a solvent used in industry in the preparation of lacquers and varnishes and was extensively used in the leather industry. It is odourless and tasteless. This chemical has been involved in a numbers of poisoning cases in which large numbers of people have been affected. However, the most notorious occurred in the USA in the 1930s. This poisoning was really a result of the conditions during prohibition which meant that people were looking for alternative ways of obtaining alcohol. One source was an alcoholic extract of Jamaica Ginger which was an official US Pharmacopoeia preparation sold for the cure of common ailments. It was allowed to be sold despite the alcohol content as the large amount of ginger it contained was believed to make it too irritating, and so unpalatable. However, adulterated versions were soon produced containing less ginger. At 35 cents a bottle, usually mixed with Coca Cola, it was drinkable and contained more alcohol than a legal drink before Prohibition. Many therefore used it as a source of alcohol. This was particularly the case amongst the poor of the southern states of the USA. However a batch of the preparation made illegally, perhaps by criminals trying to exploit the situation, was adulterated with the poisonous tri-orthocresyl phosphate. Unfortunately for the victims, the bootleggers probably used tri-orthocresyl phosphate as a solvent. The first reports appeared in 1930 and described sudden onset of cramps and sore calf muscles followed in a few hours by paralysis in both legs. The nerves affected caused the syndrome of **foot drop** which meant that those affected dragged their legs. The victims were mainly poor farmers and working class people, many of whom were out of work as this took place in the Depression and of course they were also 'drinkers'. The result was that as many as 50 000 people were poisoned and suffered permanent paralysis. In one case in Cincinnati 2500 people were affected. Those affected were both those using the preparation legitimately as well as those using it as a source of alcohol. The episode did not receive much attention probably because of the lack of political influence of those affected. Eventually twenty-one people and six corporations were indicted.

The drink was known as Ginger Jake or Jake and so the paralysis caused by the tri-orthocresylphosphate became known as **Jake Leg**. Phrases in Blues songs from that period refer to the episode:

Jake liquor, Jake liquor, what in the world you tryin' to do?
Everybody in the city messed up on account of you.
I drank so much Jake it settled all in my knee.
I reached for my loving baby but she turned her back on me.

Blues Song, 1930, Ishman Bracey

THE SPANISH OIL SYNDROME

Non-natural substances may also sometimes contaminate food and there have been several examples of this such as Epping Jaundice which has already been mentioned in Chapter 6. A more recent and tragic example of this was the contamination of cooking oil in Spain.

In May 1981 an unusual outbreak of a pulmonary disease was reported around Madrid. The unusual syndrome included severe **pulmonary oedema** which was not prolonged, **exanthema** and **eosinophilia**. Overall there were more than 20 000 cases of the syndrome and 351 fatalities (Figure 7.1). A toxic substance was suspected and finally a connection was established between the disease and the use of cheap cooking oil. Action by the Spanish Government to replace the oil with pure olive oil decreased the numbers of cases reported.

SPAIN'S POISON OIL SCANDAL

THE SUNDAY TIMES, 23 AUGUST 1981

FIGURE 7.1 *A headline reporting the disaster which followed the use of rape-seed oil contaminated with aniline as a substitute for olive oil in Spain in 1981.*
From The Sunday Times, *August 23 1981, with permission.*

There was a correlation between the consumption of cheap oil, especially that sold by certain salesmen, and the development of the syndrome.

The disease appeared after a latent period of at least 1–2 weeks, longer in some cases, and an apparent dose–response relationship was noted in one report. However, the association between the intake of oil and the syndrome is circumstantial as the effects have not been reproduced in experimental animals and the precise causative agent has not been identified. The syndrome had an acute phase with mainly acute pulmonary interstitial oedema, and a chronic phase which was mainly neuromuscular with **muscular atrophy**, **skin lesions** and **weight loss**. **Vasculitis** was also observed which affected many blood vessels.

The toxic oil was **rape-seed oil** which had been denatured by the addition of **aniline**, as required by law in Spain for imported rape seed oil so that it cannot be used for cooking. However, refining of this oil was undertaken and the resulting oil sold as suitable for human consumption. This had been practised previously without the toxic effects being seen, and consequently it seems that the particular batch of oil responsible for the syndrome may have been refined differently or was different in some other way. It was mixed with other oils in some cases and so may have become contaminated. Identifying the toxic constituents so far has not been possible. The failure to understand the mechanism underlying this major public health disaster highlights the difficulties of studying food additive/contaminant problems. These are often due to factors beyond the control of the toxicologist. In this case, the problem of obtaining samples of oil reliably associated with the syndrome and the absence of an animal model have greatly hampered the research.

This tragedy also illustrates how a large number of people may be affected by a toxic contaminant in a foodstuff. A more *subtle* toxic reaction to a food additive than the one described here could affect many *more* people before it was detected.

Summary and learning objectives

Food contains many different substances: **normal constituents**, **contaminants** and intentional **additives**. Food additives are intentionally used to colour, preserve or flavour food. Although tested for toxicity in animals, humans will be exposed for most if not all of their lives and there are indications that some additives such as **tartrazine**, a common colouring agent (E102), may lead to effects such as urticaria, perhaps in susceptible individuals. Testing additives such as the sweetener **saccharin** at high doses in animals, however, lead to pathological changes (bladder tumours) which were difficult to interpret as the kinetics are different at such high doses when elimination becomes saturated. The sweetener was banned for some time. Contaminants may result from inappropriate treatment of foodstuffs such as in the case of the **Ginger Jake** when tri-*o*-cresyl phosphate was used as solvent for ginger in a pharmaceutical preparation bought for its alcohol content as a cheap drink during Prohibition. The organophosphate caused peripheral neuropathy resulting in paralysis and foot drop ('Jake leg') in a large number of victims. In the **Spanish Oil Syndrome** contaminated rape-seed oil was sold for cooking, leading to many deaths and a large number of victims of an unusual syndrome which included muscular atrophy, weight loss and pulmonary oedema.

Contaminants such as products of mould growth may be toxic or even carcinogenic such as the aflatoxins from the mould *Aspergillus flavus* which grows on crops such as peanuts. Aflatoxin B_1 causes liver cancer as a result of metabolic activation and interaction of the metabolite with DNA. Others may be produced by bacterial contaminating food such as *Salmonella* or *Clostridium botulinum*.

Questions

Q1. Match the following food additives with the appropriate category.

Erythrosine	Flavour enhancer
Monosodium glutamate	Anti-oxidant
Cinnamaldehyde	Colouring agent
Butylated hydroxytoluene	Bleach
Benzoyl peroxide	Flavour

Q2. Indicate which of the following is true or false?
Tartrazine:

a   is a flavouring agent
b   may cause urticaria
c   is reduced by gut bacteria
d   is known as F102
c   is a derivative of aspirin.

Q3. Indicate which of the following is true or false?
The sweetener saccharin:

a   causes bladder tumours in rats at high doses
b   was discovered by Delaney et al
c   is banned for use as a sweetener worldwide
d   has low acute toxicity
e   shows saturation pharmacokinetics.

Q4. Indicate which are true or false?
     The Spanish oil syndrome:

    a   was caused by the use of adulterated
        sunflower oil for cooking
    b   was caused by tri-orthocresyl phos-
        phate used in cooking
    c   is a type of muscular dystrophy
    d   causes pulmonary oedema.

SHORT ANSWER QUESTION

Q5. Name three naturally occuring toxicants
     and briefly explain where and how they
     arise in food.

Bibliography

Casarett and Doull's Toxicology, The Basic Science of Poisons, C. D. Klaassen (Ed.), 5th edition, 1996, New York: McGraw-Hill. Various chapters.

General and Applied Toxicology, Ballantyne, B., Marrs, T. and Syversen, T. L. M. (Eds), 2nd edition, 1999, Basingstoke: Macmillan. Various chapters.

HANSSEN, M. and MARSDEN, J. (1984) *E for Additives,* Wellingborough: Thorsons.

JUHLIN, L. (1983) Intolerance to food and drug additives, in *Allergic Reactions to Drugs,* de Weck, A. L. and Bundgaard, H. (Eds), Berlin: Springer Verlag.

LIN, J-K. and HO, Y-S. (1994) Hepatotoxic Actions of Dietary Amines. *Toxicology and Ecotoxicology News,* **1**, 82-87.

MILLER, K. and NICKLIN, S. (1984) Adverse reactions to food additives and colours, in *Developments in Food Colours,* vol. 2, Walford, J. (Ed.), Amsterdam: Elsevier Applied Science.

NAS (1978) Saccharin: Technical Assessment of Risks and Benefits, Report No. 1, Washington, DC: Committee for a Study on Saccharin and Food Safety Policy.

RECHCIGL, M. (Ed.) (1983) *Handbook of Naturally Occurring Food Toxicants,* Boca Raton: CRC Press.

World Health Organisation (1984) Toxic Oil Syndrome, Report on a WHO Meeting, Madrid 1983, Copenhagen: WHO.

CHAPTER — 8

Pesticides

Chapter outline

In this chapter the toxicity of different types of pesticides will be studied:

- Introduction and types of pesticides
- DDT
- Organophosphorus compounds
- Paraquat
- Fluoroacetate

Introduction

Pesticides are substances which have been designed or chosen for selective toxicity to certain organisms. Although their toxicity *is* selective, they are often also toxic to other species although usually to a *lesser* degree. As well as being of interest in terms of their mode of action they are of concern to toxicologists for two reasons: **(1)** they may be **toxic to man** either in acute poisonings or after **chronic exposure**; and **(2)** they have toxic effects on some **non-target organisms** in the environment. This latter point was highlighted in 1963 by Rachel Carson in her book *Silent Spring*.

Human poisonings from accidental exposure to pesticides have occurred since they were first used and in some cases many people have been poisoned, sometimes fatally in single incidents. Many of these cases have been due to accidental contamination of food with pesticides or their inappropriate use (Table 8.1). For example, the use of organic **mercury fungicides** to treat seed grain which is then used to feed animals has resulted in several mass poisonings of humans. Occupational poisoning has also occurred in agricultural workers through accidental contamination or inappropriate use. The careless use of pesticides, such as spraying without adequate protection, may also lead to exposure of the operator.

Chronic toxicity due to the pesticides present in our environment is more difficult to identify although with the development of improved analytical techniques the detection of residues has become easier. Such techniques have

TABLE 8.1 *Mass poisonings due to pesticides*

Pesticide involved	Material contaminated	Number affected	(died)	Location
Endrin	Flour	159	(0)	Wales
Endrin	Flour	691	(24)	Qatar
Parathion	Flour	600	(88)	Colombia
Parathion	Sugar	300	(17)	Mexico
Hexachlorobenzene	Seed grain	>3000	(3–11%)	Turkey
Organic mercury	Seed grain	321	(35)	Iraq
Pentachlorophenol	Nursery linens	20	(2)	USA

Source: *Report of the Secretary's Commission on Pesticides and Their Relationship to Environmental Health* (Washington, DC: US Governmental Printing Office, 1969).

shown that most people in the Western World are indeed exposed to and may have detectable levels of certain pesticides. However, pesticides have become a very important part of our society especially in terms of agricultural economics and, although their use may be curtailed in some instances, it is unlikely to be completely halted when risk/benefit considerations are made.

Pesticides can be divided into several groups, such as **insecticides, fungicides, herbicides** and **rodenticides**, depending on the target organism. Those that have been specifically designed for a purpose often utilize a particular biological, metabolic or other feature of the target species, but unfortunately such features are *rarely entirely unique* to that species so other similar species may also be affected. A simple example of selective toxicity in a pesticide is the use of **warfarin** as a rodenticide. This depends on the *lack* of the vomit reflex in rats so that they are unable to vomit after ingesting the poison.

Other pesticides depend on more sophisticated biochemical differences. For example, the insecticide **malathion** is metabolized by *hydrolysis* in mammals to yield the acidic metabolite, which is readily excreted (Figure 3.9). In insects, however, the preferred metabolic route is *oxidation* to yield **malaoxon** which is toxic by inhibition of **cholinesterase** (see below). Although pesticides may all be perceived by the general public as equally hazardous to man, they vary in their toxicity to mammals, and other non-target wildlife, and in their effects on the environment

Some examples of the major pesticide types are as follows:

Insecticides: Organophosphorus compounds, carbamate and organochlorine compounds. Natural products such as pyrethrins.

Herbicides: Chlorophenoxy compounds, dinitrophenols, bipyridyls, carbamates, triazines, substituted ureas, aromatic amides.

Fungicides: alkyl mercury compounds, chlorinated hydrocarbons, dialkyldithiocarbamates, organotin compounds.

Rodenticides: inorganic agents, natural products, fluorinated aliphatics, α-naphthylthiourea.

It is clear from this list that pesticides comprise a wide range of chemical types and their modes of action will be very different. However, their toxicity to man and other mammals may be due to a different mechanism from their pesticidal action.

We will now consider some toxicologically important examples of pesticides.

DDT

Perhaps the best known organochlorine insecticide is DDT, (dichloro-diphenyl-trichloroethane; Figure 8.1). It was introduced in 1945 for the control of **malarial mosquitoes** and was extremely successful, being a major factor in the reduction in malaria after the Second World War. DDT is a contact poison which is highly potent against the insect nervous system but is relatively non-toxic to man. A dose of at least 10 mg kg^{-1} is required for toxic effects to occur in man and no human fatalities have been reported. Indeed human volunteers were induced to take 0.5 mg kg^{-1} (35 mg) daily for over a year and there was no demonstrable toxicity. Although some reports have suggested association between chronic disease and DDT, no causal relationship has been found and other reports have not found such associations. Large doses cause **tremors, hyperexcitability** and **convulsions, paresthesias, irritability** and **dizziness**. In experimental animals liver damage occurs after single large doses and **hypertrophy** and other histological changes in **liver** have been reported after chronic exposure. Toxic effects seem mainly to involve the nervous system in mammals as in insects. The mechanism of action is unknown but the primary site of action is thought to be sensory; **motor nerve fibres** and the **motor cortex** are possible targets. DDT may alter *transport* of Na$^+$ and K$^+$ across nerve membranes perhaps by interfering with the energy metabolism required for this transport.

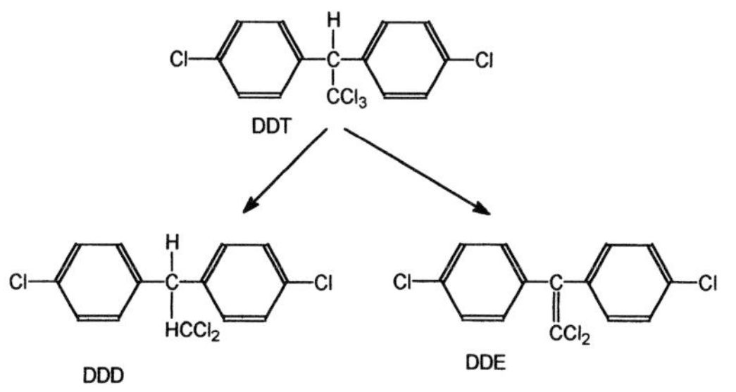

DDT is chemically stable, highly insoluble in water, but soluble in body fat and is consequently very persistent in biological systems and the environment (Table 8.2). It is poorly absorbed through the skin and is metabolized in animals by a number of routes (Figure 8.1) but the metabolite DDE is more persistent than the parent compound (Table 8.2). There are other metabolites such as an acidic derivative which is more water-soluble but the conversion to these is slow and does not involve major routes. There are also microbial and environmental degradation to other metabolites.

FIGURE 8.1 *Two of the pathways of metabolism of the insecticide dichloro-diphenyl-trichloroethane (DDT).*

TABLE 8.2 *Persistence of the insecticide DDT and its metabolites*

Compound	Half-life in pigeon (days)	Half-life in soil (yrs)
DDT	28	2.5–5
DDD	23	
DDE	250	

It is because of this persistence, that DDT levels in the environment have been increasing ever since it was first used. Furthermore, the DDT concentration in some of the exposed organisms increases at each higher trophic level of the **food chain** (see Chapter 9). For example, small organisms such as plankton or *Daphnia* absorb DDT passively or via filter feeding from river or lake water and this enters their body fat. The concentration in the tissues of these organisms may be several hundred or thousand fold greater than the concentration in the surrounding water. Then, either insects or small fish eat these small organisms and the DDT is transferred to their fat tissue (Table 8.3). These small organisms are in turn eaten by still larger organisms and so on up the food chain. As DDT is fat soluble it remains in the organism and is then transferred into the fat of the predator or animal at the top of the food chain which may be man. The result is that relatively high concentrations of DDT can occur in those animals at the top of the food chain by a continuous process of amplification or **biomagnification** despite the fact that the initial concentration of DDT in the water is low. This is illustrated by the following example: in one area of California, plankton were found to contain 4 ppm of DDT, while the bass found in the same area contained 138 ppm and the grebes feeding on them 1500 ppm. So what seems to be a negligible concentration of DDT in the river or lake water or at the bottom of a food chain may be biologically very significant at the top. Toxic concentrations of DDT appear to affect birds and fish particularly in the production of eggs. It can be shown, for example, that there is a relationship between shell thickness and DDE concentration in birds of prey such as the kestrel (Figure 8.2).

In man, as in other animals exposed to DDT, most is located in the body **fat**. The concentration in fat is proportional to the intake, reaching a plateau with a half-life of around six months. The estimated intake for humans in the USA was around 35 mg year^{-1} in 1969 but the level in food is declining as is the amount in human fat. The acceptable yearly intake for humans as given by the **FAO/WHO guidelines** is 255 mg year^{-1}. The DDT either comes from eating food of animal origin where the animal itself or another lower in the food chain has been exposed, or from vegetables or fruit

TABLE 8.3 *Example of a food chain*

Organism	Tropic Level
Pine trees	1st Producers
Aphids	2nd Herbivores
Spiders	3rd Insectivores
Tits and Warblers	4th Insectivores
Hawks	5th Carnivores

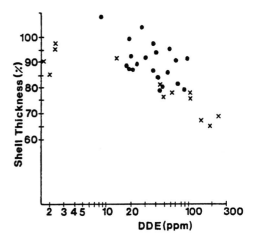

FIGURE 8.2 *The relationship between shell thickness and residues of the DDT metabolite DDE. The data is from kestrel eggs collected in Ithaca, New York in 1970 (●) or experimentally induced with dietary DDE (X). The data is the mean clutch thickness expressed as percent of control egg thickness collected before DDT use. Data from Lincer, J. L. (1975),* Journal of Applied Ecology, *12, 781.*

which have been sprayed or otherwise con-taminated.

The DDT in fat does not appear to be harm-ful to animals, however, and there is no correla-tion between adipose tissue levels and signs of poisoning. It is the concentration circulating in the **blood** which is more relevant to the toxic effects, and more particularly the level in the brain. However, if there is a reduction of the fat content of the body, the blood level will *rise*. Experiments with rats have shown that this increase in blood level can lead to toxicity. It has been found recently that bats in the south-ern USA have high levels of DDT even though it is no longer used. This is probably because the bats eat large quantities of insects and there is sufficient *residual* DDT in the environment for it to appear in **food chains**. In a particular spe-cies of bat this has been a problem because the DDT is passed via the milk to young bats and this then enters their fat tissues. When the bats go on mass long-distance migration, they start to mobilize this fat and so their blood levels of DDT increase until they become sufficient to cause toxicity and death.

Human milk may also contain **DDT** and as with other food chains there is a concentration effect. For example, lactating mothers exposed to 0.0005 mg kg^{-1} day^{-1} were found to pro-duce milk containing 0.08 ppm DDT, hence their infants were exposed to 0.0112 mg kg^{-1} day^{-1}, an exposure some twenty times greater than the mothers.

There is no real evidence that DDT under such chronic exposure conditions is overtly toxic in man although there is some evidence that it is carcinogenic in mice. Consequently continuous exposure to low levels of DDT may constitute a long-term hazard. Chronic exposure to DDT does lead to induction of the microsomal enzymes involved in the meta-bolism of foreign compounds. It may be this effect that causes the **hormonal imbalance**

seen in birds, as some hormones are also meta-bolized by the microsomal enzymes.

The story of DDT illustrates the problems of using chemicals in our environment and the assessment of risks and benefits. DDT is a very cheap and effective insecticide. Unfortunately it was used rather indiscrimi-nately in agriculture in the USA in the early years after its introduction. The result of this was a marked decrease in the wild bird popula-tion. This was presumably partly due to the decrease in the number of insects on which the birds fed but was also a result of the direct toxic effect of DDT on the birds themselves. Improvements in analytical techniques allowed residues of DDT to be easily detected in many of the carcasses of the dead birds and other animals found.

These findings were meticulously documen-ted by an American zoologist, Rachel Carson and published in her book *Silent Spring*. The book became a bestseller and consequently DDT was soon a notorious pollutant and was banned from use in many countries. The assumption was made that if this substance was responsible for such devastating effects on birds and other wildlife it must be bad for humans. However, this story illustrates a num-ber of important points.

1   The finding that the carcasses of birds and other animals contained detectable levels of DDT does not prove that this was the cause of death.

2   DDT can be detected at very low concentra-tions in biological samples with sophisti-cated analytical techniques but this does not mean that such concentrations are dangerous or poisonous.

3   Birds are very different creatures to humans and other mammals.

DDT is very toxic to insects and consequently it is used as an insecticide but insect biochemistry and physiology is also different from that in humans.

The problems arose with DDT because of the indiscriminate use of the insecticide in agriculture. If it had been used more carefully then the problems with the wildlife might not have occurred. There have been two effects of banning DDT:

a   Other insecticides have been developed and used and many of them are much more toxic to mammals than DDT and some have resulted in a significant number of human deaths.

b   The control of the malarial mosquito for which DDT is very effective has been hampered and hence malaria is still prevalent in some parts of the world.

Furthermore, it should be noted that DDT has not been responsible for a single human death and there is very little evidence that it is toxic in humans.

The risk–benefit argument therefore is that the benefits of DDT used *responsibly* for the control of *disease-carrying* insects far outweigh the risks to humans. Unfortunately, misuse and public hysteria have clouded the rational scientific arguments.

Most other organochlorine insecticides such as **heptachlor**, **gamma-HCH**, **dieldrin** and **aldrin**, have similar problems of persistence to DDT.

Organophosphorus compounds

The use of organochlorine insecticides has decreased recently because of their persistence and because of fears about their long-term effects. The case against DDT is mainly due to its environmental impact on wildlife rather than its toxicity to man, which seems to be low. However, the organophosphorus compounds which have replaced the organochlorine type of insecticide are often *more toxic* to mammals (maybe as much as one hundred times more toxic), if less persistent.

There have been a significant number of human poisonings from organophosphorus compounds which are the major cause of poisonings in agricultural workers in California.

Case study   *In Pakistan in 1976 in a programme to eradicate malarial mosquitoes a significant number of workers using **malathion** suffered poisoning (2800 out of 7500 sprayers) and there were five deaths. The malathion was used as a water dispersable powder. The components of the powder and the storage caused the malathion to change. The temperature was too high in some storage facilities and some of the malathion was converted into iso-malathion. This contaminant then made the malathion very much more toxic in the exposed humans.*

There are many organophosphorus compounds now used as insecticides and their mode of action and toxicity is similar. As already indicated organophosphorus compounds are more toxic and have been responsible for more human deaths and illness than the organochlorine type of pesticide. **Parathion**, first synthesized in 1944 (Figure 8.3), is one widely used organophosphorus insecticide which has featured in a number of documented **mass human poisonings** (Table 8.1) and probably in many isolated incidents. Parathion has high mammalian toxicity and consequently it has been superseded by other less toxic organophosphorus compounds for certain uses. One such insecticide is **malathion** (Figure 3.9) which is more **selective** in its **toxi-**

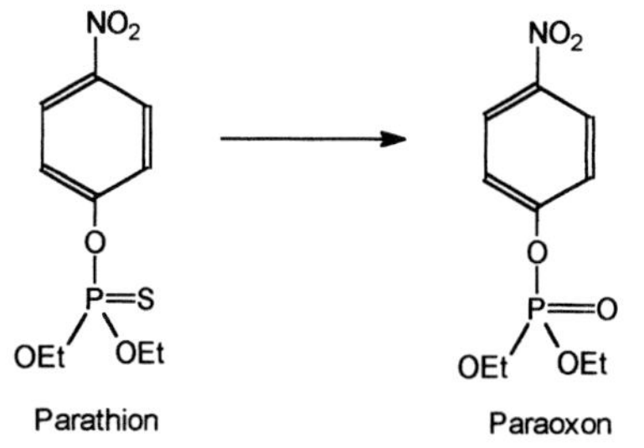

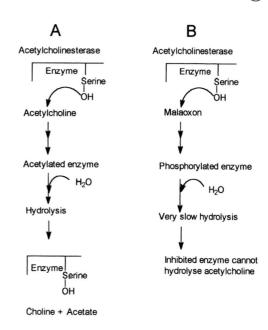

FIGURE 8.3 *The oxidative metabolism of the insecticide parathion.*
From Timbrell, J. A., Principles of Biochemical Toxicology, *Taylor & Francis, London, 1991.*

FIGURE 8.4 *The mechanisms of hydrolysis of acetylcholine by acetylcholinesterase (A) and the interaction of the malathion metabolite malaoxon with the enzyme (B).*

city mainly because of differences in its metabolism between mammals and insects. However, the effects of organophosphorus compounds are qualitatively similar and can be considered collectively.

Poisoning with organophosphorus compounds is an example of an **exaggerated pharmacological effect** rather than of direct toxic action and the toxicity may be either *cumulative* following chronic exposure or acute after a single exposure. Organophosphorus compounds exert their toxicity by interfering with the enzyme **acetylcholinesterase**. The organophosphorus compound binds to this enzyme because of similarities with the natural substrate for the enzyme, a neurotransmitter present in the nervous system called **acetylcholine**. Once its job at nerve endings is done, acetylcholine is hydrolysed by the enzyme, acetylcholinesterase and so removed. This terminates the action of the acetylcholine as a chemical transmitter at nerve endings. However, organophosphorus compounds inhibit this enzyme and so the acetylcholine accumulates leading to excessive stimulation of the nerve (Figure 8.4). This will lead to the death of the insect.

The same will occur in humans and other mammalian species. However, the organophosphorus insecticides have been devised so that the metabolism is different in mammals from insects and the organophosphorus compounds

are detoxified in mammals. However, this is only efficient at low exposure levels and at higher levels humans will suffer the same consequences as insects. In the case of the poisoning in Pakistan, it was the alternative, detoxication route of metabolism, which was inhibited by the impurity and so the humans exposed became, like insects, much more susceptible.

Various different types of organophosphorus compounds inhibit cholinesterase enzymes and so cause a spectrum of similar toxic effects. These include headaches, nightmares, salivation and increased tear formation, diarrhoea and constriction of the passages in the lungs. These symptoms are all due to the increased levels of *acetylcholine*. Depending on the particular organophosphorus compound the inhibition may be *reversible* or *irreversible*. The **acetylcholinesterases** in different tissues such as plasma and nerves are different and so are not equally inhibited by organophosphorus compounds. There are degrees of inhibition of the total body acetylcholinesterase; in mammals a level of 50 per cent inhibition leads to toxic effects and 80–90 per cent inhibition will be lethal. The mechanism of toxicity of organophosphorus compounds relies on their similarity to the normal substrate **acetylcholine** (Figure 8.4). Thus, the organophosphorus compound is also a substrate for the enzyme but unlike acetylcholine, the product remains bound to the active site and the resulting complex may be only *slowly hydrolyzed*, if at all. With those organophosphorus compounds causing *irreversible inhibition*, resynthesis of the enzyme is necessary.

Malathion itself is not a substrate for cholinesterases but requires metabolism to **malaoxon**. This takes place readily in insects but in mammals hydrolysis is the preferred route and this leads to a readily excreted diacid (Figure 3.9). This is the basis of the selective toxicity.

The toxic effects of organophosphorus compounds centre around the *excessive* cholinergic stimulation with death occurring a a result of **neuromuscular paralysis** and **central depression**. Some organophosphorus compounds also cause another toxic effect where the nerves in the arms and legs die. This is known as **peripheral neuropathy** and the result is paralysis. However, not all organophosphorus compounds cause this and it is unrelated to the ability to inhibit the enzyme cholinesterase. One particular organophosphorus compound, **triorthocresyl phosphate** (TOCP), is a very potent agent in causing this effect. It is used in industry as a solvent. However, there have been a number of large-scale poisoning episodes generally in relation to food and these will be discussed under **Food additives and contaminants** (see above).

Paraquat

The examples mentioned so far have been insecticides which, as a group, are probably more important than other pesticides in terms of human and environmental toxicity. However, one particular **herbicide** is of particular importance and notoriety in terms of human toxicology. This is paraquat (Figure 8.5) which, during the more than twenty years of its use, has featured in several hundred cases of **fatal human poisoning**. Unlike the organophosphorus compounds, however, this has not been the result of accidental contamination of food and unlike the organochlorines there has been no particular environmental impact. Paraquat poisoning has mainly been the result of deliberate ingestion, usually orally, for **suicide** or **murder** with a few cases of **accidental** direct ingestion. Paraquat is a contact herbicide which binds very strongly to soil. Consequently it does not leach out of soil after being sprayed onto plants and does not have an environmental effect either on other plants or animals. Paraquat kills the plant by interfering with photosynthesis and its toxicity to animals may have some similarities at the biochemical level. When ingested by humans paraquat is usually fatal but even if it is not it may cause **serious lung and kidney damage**. The lung is the target organ because it *selectively* accumulates paraquat and consequently the concentration in the alveolar type I and II

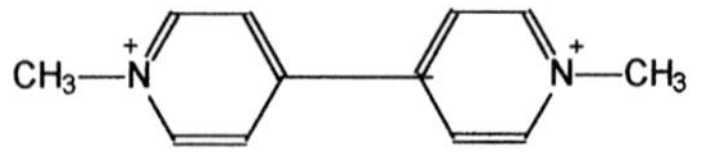

FIGURE 8.5 *The structure of the herbicide paraquat (A), and the polyamines putrescine (B) and spermine (C).*

lung cells reaches sufficient levels to cause toxic effects in those cells. The concentration in the lungs reaches a level *several times* that in the plasma and the paraquat is retained in the lung even when the plasma concentration is falling. Paraquat is taken up by the lung because of a structural similarity with **diamines** and **polyamines**, such as **putrescine**, **spermine** and **spermidine** (Figure 8.5). The presence of two nitrogens in paraquat, with a particular intramolecular distance, enables paraquat, but not the herbicide **diquat**, to be taken up by a selective active transport system in the lung for which polyamines are the normal substrate. The only other organ with an uptake system for polyamines is the brain which does not seem to accumulate paraquat.

Paraquat is believed to cause toxicity via its **free radical** form which is stable and results from an enzyme-mediated, one electron *reduction* which requires NADPH (Figure 8.6). In the presence of oxygen this generates **superoxide anion** and the paraquat cation reforms. This redox cycling continues to produce superoxide and deplete NADPH. The superoxide can lead to the production of **hydrogen peroxide** and **hydroxyl radicals**. Hydroxyl radicals are highly reactive and can cause **lipid peroxidation** which in turn causes further metabolic disruption. The presence of oxygen in the lungs is clearly an important factor in the pathogenesis of the lung lesion. The toxicity to the lungs is a direct result of the distribution of paraquat as the active uptake into lung cells gives rise to the relatively high and toxic concentration.

Paraquat causes a progressive **fibrosis** of the lungs and also damages the kidneys; once absorbed there is no antidote. The only treatments available are either an attempt to limit absorption by oral administration of substances such as **Fullers Earth** which *adsorb* paraquat or the use of **haemodialysis** or **haemoperfusion** to rid the blood of the paraquat. After the paraquat has accumulated in the lungs, however, there is no effective treatment currently available.

Paraquat has been used on many occasions for suicide and parasuicide attempts but unfortunately for the victim death is slow and painful,

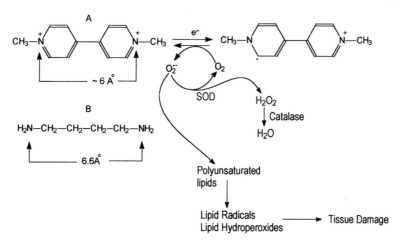

FIGURE 8.6 *The proposed mechanism for the lung toxicity of paraquat. The paraquat molecule, (A), readily forms a free radical by accepting an electron from cellular donors such as NADPH. The paraquat radical donates its unpaired electron to oxygen forming superoxide, which is reactive. It is detoxified by superoxide dismutase (SOD), but in excessive amounts overloads the enzyme and causes lipid peroxidation, leading to tissue damage. Paraquat has similarities to putrescine, (B), having two nitrogen atoms a similar distance apart. Therefore paraquat is a substrate for the putrescine active uptake system in the lung and so is accumulated there.*

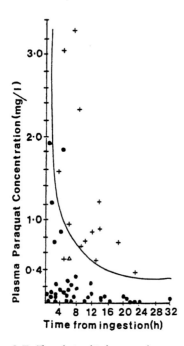

FIGURE 8.7   *The relationship between plasma paraquat concentration and the outcome of the poisoning, death (+) or survival (●). Δ is an aspiration death.*
Data from Vale, J. A. and Meredith, T. J., Paraquat Poisoning, pp. 135–141, Figure 21.4 in Poisoning – Diagnosis and Treatment, *Vale, J. A. and Meredith, T. J., (Eds) Update Books, London, 1981.*

occurring over a period of several days to a week or more with the progressive fibrosis of the lung leading to eventual suffocation. The prognosis is usually bad and the plasma level of paraquat indicates the likely outcome (Figure 8.7).

Fluoroacetate

Monofluoroacetate is an interesting example of a pesticide which is also a **natural product**. This compound is highly toxic by virtue of its very specific blockade of Krebs (tricarboxylic acid) cycle. Fluoroacetate is a **pseudosubstrate** and is successfully incorporated into Krebs cycle as **fluoroacetyl CoA**. The **fluorocitrate** produced will bind to the enzyme **aconitase**, but after binding the pseudosubstrate, the enzyme cannot remove the fluorine atom and so the enzyme is *blocked*. Therefore, Krebs cycle is unable to function and the cell and organism dies through lack of metabolic intermediates and energy.

Fluoroacetate is found naturally in some plants in Australia, Africa and South America. Some indigenous animals in Australia, especially the skink and emu have developed tolerance. However, introduced and unadapted animals, such as rats, mice, cats and dogs and those living outside the areas where fluoroacetate producing plants grow, are more susceptible to fluoroacetate toxicity (see Twigg and King, 1991). This is an example of what has been termed '**chemical warfare**' between plants and animals. The plants produce such toxic substances to stop animals eating them. However, fluoroacetate is also used as a pesticide for example in New Zealand, where it is known as **1080** and is used to kill **possums** which have become pests.

Summary and learning objectives

Pesticides are chemicals that have been *specifically designed* to be toxic and generally lethal to a particular organism such as an *insect, plant, fungus* or *rodent*. Some pesticides show *selective toxicity* and only damage the target organ but others are less selective and therefore are toxic to non-target organisms, including man. The widespread and initially rather indiscriminate use of the insecticide *DDT* causing the death of large numbers of birds and other wildlife led to it being banned in a number of countries. Although relatively non-toxic to mammals, DDT is a very effective insecticide for the control of the malarial mosquito. Insect nerve fibres are the biochemical target. DDT and its metabolites are lipophilic and undergo bioaccumulation in the food chain. Consequently, those animals at the top of that chain such as birds may be exposed to higher concentrations of the pesticide. The destruction of non-target insects also reduces the natural food supply. Toxicity, especially chronic toxicity due to pesticides in mammals such as man has occurred, particularly from those pesticides that replaced DDT such as the **organophosphates** (e.g. parathion, malathion). These act by inhibiting acetyl-cholinesterase, usually after metabolic transformation. However, in mammals, alternative detoxication pathways may be available. Inhibition of acetylcholinesterase may be irreversible and in mammals leads to accumulation of acetylcholine, which causes toxic effects which include salivation, diarrhoea, bronchoconstriction and respiratory failure. Some organophosphates (e.g. TOCP) also cause peripheral neuropathy. Pesticides may be highly toxic to humans, such as the herbicide **paraquat**, which causes lung damage as a result of selective uptake and accumulation in lung cells and production of reactive oxygen species. Natural pesticides also exist such as the highly toxic plant product **fluoroacetate**, which blocks Krebs' cycle and is lethal to mammals as a result of heart failure, except those wild species that have developed tolerance.

Questions

Q1. Indicate which are true or false. DDT:

   a   is an organophosphate
   b   is very lipid soluble

   c   is toxic to mammals
   d   is metabolized by loss of HCl
   e   inhibits cholinesterase
   f   is a herbicide
   g   is toxic to eggs.

Q2. Indicate which are true or false. Parathion is an insecticide which:

   a   has low toxicity to humans
   b   is not metabolized
   c   acts by inhibiting Na K ATPase
   d   causes excessive cholinergic stimulation
   e   causes bronchoconstriction.

Q3. Indicate which are true or false. Paraquat:

   a   is an organochlorine insecticide
   b   is metabolized to diquat by SOD
   c   causes lipid peroxidation
   d   is concentrated in lung tissue
   e   causes liver fibrosis
   f   blocks uptake of putrescine into the brain.

SHORT ANSWER QUESTION

Q4. What is the underlying basis of fluoroacetate toxicity?

Bibliography

ALDRIDGE, W. N. (1996) *Mechanisms and Concepts in Toxicology*, London: Taylor & Francis.

ECHOBICHON, D. J. (Ed.) (1998) *Occupational Hazards of Pesticide Exposure: Sampling, Monitoring, Measuring*, Washington: Hemisphere.

HAYES, W. J. (1975) *Toxicology of Pesticides*, Baltimore: Waverley Press.

HAYES, W. J. (1982) *Pesticides Studied in Man*, Baltimore: Williams and Wilkins.

MATSUMURA, F. (1975) *Toxicology of Insecticides,* New York: Plenum Press.

MORIATY, F. (1999) *Ecotoxicology: The Study of Pollutants in Ecosystems*, 3rd edition, London: Academic Press.

RAND, G.M. (Ed.), (1995) *Fundamentals of Aquatic Toxicology*, Taylor & Francis. A large, comprehensive text.

SHAW, I. C. and CHADWICK, J. (1998) *Principles of Environmental Toxicology*, London: Taylor & Francis.

TWIGG, L. E. and KING, D. R. (1991) The impact of fluoroacetate-bearing vegetation on native Australian fauna: a review. *Oikos*, **61**: 412–430.

WALKER, C. H., HOPKIN, S. P., SIBLY, R. M. and PEAKALL, D. B. (2001) *Principles of Ecotoxicology*, 2nd edition, London: Taylor & Francis.

CHAPTER — **9**

Environmental pollutants

Chapter outline

This chapter examines the various aspects of environmental pollution and explores some specific examples:

- Introduction
- Air pollution
- Particulates
- Acid rain
- Lead pollution
- Water pollution
- Arsenic
- Food chains
- Endocrine disruptors
- Mercury and methylmercury

Introduction

Pollution of our environment has become an increasing problem over the last century with the development of industry and agriculture and with the increase in population. That is not to say that pollution did not exist before the nineteenth century, indeed there was legislation enacted in Britain during the thirteenth century to control smoke from household fires in London. However, pollution on the current scale started during the **Industrial Revolution**. Nineteenth-century factories used coal for fuel and in certain processes, and consequently smoke was a major pollutant. Blast furnaces and chemical plants added other fumes and other types of noxious substance. As many industrial processes used water for power, as part of the process, or in some other way, factories were often sited near rivers and effluent was discharged into them. In this way both the atmosphere and rivers became polluted. More recently the land has also become polluted from agricultural use of fertilizers and pesticides, as well as from the dumping of toxic wastes from factories and industrial processes. Consequently air, water and the earth have all suffered pollution and we may divide environmental pollution into these categories.

Despite the appalling working and living conditions which existed during the Industrial Revolution in parts of Britain during the nineteenth century and in heavily industrialized areas in other European countries and the USA, it was not until the twentieth century that a serious attempt was made to curb pollution. One event which precipitated this was the **'great smog' in London** in the winter of **1952**. A combination of weather conditions and smoke from domestic coal fires, factories and power stations resulted in a thick smog which contributed to the deaths of over *four thousand* people (Figure 9.1).

At around the same time the River Thames was found to be so highly polluted that fish, particularly salmon, could not live in the lower parts of the river. This was as a result of industrial processes and other processes dumping effluent into the river. The same was true in some other cities in the UK and in other industrial countries.

In Britain, as a result of the smog, the Clean Air Act was passed which led to a reduction in the production of smoke in cities. Other legislation concerned with pollution of rivers allowed the gradual clean-up of the Thames. Now smogs in London no longer occur and there are salmon swimming in the Thames. This has taken many years, however, and in other parts of Britain, as in some other countries, clean-up of the environment has not always been so successful. Air pollution from coal-burning power stations still occurs and it is now recognized that this pollution travels many hundreds of miles from countries such as Britain to Norway, Sweden and Germany, and from the USA to Canada. In these countries the air pollutants and acid rain (see page 125) cause damage to trees and other plant life and also to fish and other aquatic organisms. This illustrates that pollution is an *international* rather than a purely national problem.

Pollution of the environment is usually a continuous, deliberate process although industrial and other accidents may also contribute to environmental pollution in an acute rather than chronic manner. Let us consider some examples of environmental pollution.

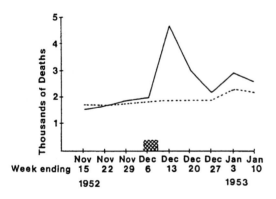

FIGURE 9.1 *Deaths associated with the London 'fog' of December 1952. The solid curve shows the number of weekly deaths in Greater London before and after the 'fog' whereas the dotted line shows the average number of deaths for the preceding 5 years. The hatched area shows the dates of the 'fog'.*
Data from Goldsmith, J. R. in Air Pollution, *Vol. 1. Chapter 10, pp. 335–386, Figure 1. Ed. A. C. Stern, NY: Academic Press, 1962.*

Air pollution

The study of air pollution involves many disciplines ranging from chemistry, engineering, epidemiology, zoology, botany, ecology, toxicology and meteorology to economics and politics. It is not a new phenomenon although it has only relatively recently become of such importance.

The most visible form of air pollution is of course **smoke** but this contains many constituents depending on the source and is accompanied by various potentially **toxic gases**. The burning of the fossil fuels coal and oil as well as certain industrial processes give rise to the gases **sulphur dioxide**, **carbon dioxide**, **carbon monoxide** and **nitrogen oxides**, and perhaps **hydrogen sulphide**, **volatile hydrocarbons**, and **particulate matter** such as carbon and ash. In Britain these amount to millions of tonnes per year; sulphur dioxide from burning fuel amounts to at least 4 million tonnes discharged into the atmosphere every year. In the USA the five major pollutants which amount to 98 per cent of all the air pollution are carbon monoxide (52 per cent), sulphur oxides (18 per cent), hydrocarbons (12 per cent), particulates (10 per cent) and nitrogen oxides (6 per cent). These air pollutants arise from the combustion of fuels in **power stations** and domestically, from **car exhausts**, from **industrial processes**, and from **waste disposal**.

The composition and dispersion of air pollutants may also be influenced by climatic conditions and can lead to 'smog'. Originally this term was coined to describe the combination of fog and smoke which hung over industrial cities under damp atmospheric conditions but it now also includes air pollution from car exhausts which has been modified by climatic conditions.

There are in fact two types of smog. **(1) Reducing smog** which has a high level of particulates and sulphur dioxide and comes from coal burning in particular. It results from a combination of incomplete combustion, fog and cool temperatures. **(2) Photochemical-oxidant smog**, for which Los Angeles is notorious, has a high concentration of ozone, nitrogen oxides and hydrocarbons. This is an oxidizing pollutant mixture arising particularly from the interaction of the constituents of car exhausts in bright sunlight.

Meteorologic inversion, as occurs in the Los Angeles basin, not only promotes this interaction but also traps the pollutants near the ground. The constituents of air pollution may in turn be altered in the atmosphere. For example, hydrogen sulphide and nitrogen dioxide may be oxidized to sulphuric and nitric acids respectively.

Ozone arises from a cyclic reaction between nitrogen dioxide and oxygen, with ultraviolet light and hydrocarbons as necessary catalysts:

$$NO_2 \overset{uv}{\rightarrow} NO + O$$
$$O_2 + O \rightarrow O_3$$
$$O_3 + NO \rightarrow NO_2 + O_2$$

What are the effects of all these pollutants on the health of man and the animals and plants in the environment?

Some of the acute effects on human health are known from several episodes which have occurred within the last 50 years. The three major episodes which have led to increased human mortality and morbidity were in the **Meuse Valley** in Belgium (1930), in **Donora**, Pennsylvania (1948), and in **London** (1952). In each case the area was heavily polluted and the same meteorological conditions (inversion) prevailed which allowed a stagnant mass of polluted air to accumulate and the pollution level to rise.

Sixty-five people died in Belgium and twenty in Donora. *Four thousand* deaths in London were attributed to the smog (Figure 9.1). These deaths were mainly in elderly people who already had respiratory or cardiac disease. After the smog in Belgium it had been predicted that a similar occurrence in London would lead to 3200 extra deaths. In fact there were 4000. On the worst day of the smog, the daily average pollutant levels were: **sulphur dioxide** 1.34 ppm and **smoke** 4.5 mg m^{-3}. Another London smog in 1962 resulted in

400 extra deaths. It has been estimated that a sulphur dioxide level of 0.25 ppm and a smoke level of 0.75 mg m^{-3} will produce an increase in mortality over the normal rate. Epidemiological studies of human populations have shown a higher incidence of **pulmonary** and **cardiovascular disease** in association with smog. Air pollution is believed to be a factor in lung cancer, the incidence of which is higher in urban areas but there are many unknown and possibly confounding factors. Some correlation has also been detected between certain other diseases, such as heart disease, with pollution levels. Chronic air pollution certainly aggravates existing respiratory diseases including the common cold and may even be a contributory factor. Filtration of air gives relief to some susceptible individuals. One early study in Britain showed a striking correlation between levels of certain pollutants (the reducing type) and the level of discomfort of patients with chronic bronchitis. It was estimated that the levels of smoke and sulphur dioxide needed to be below 0.25 mg m^{-3} and 0.19 ppm respectively for there to be no response. Indeed, the mortality from chronic bronchitis is correlated with the amount of sulphur dioxide and dust levels.

There is, however, less data on the effects of photochemical-oxidant pollution on human health. One study examined the performance of an athletic team in Los Angeles in the USA over several seasons and monitored photochemical-oxidant pollutant levels. There was a *striking correlation* between the level of oxidizing pollutants in the air and a decrease in performance, with effects demonstrated at a level as low as 0.1 ppm. The mean oxidant level in Los Angeles at this time exceeded 0.1 ppm and the maximum hourly level reached 0.6 ppm at certain times. Lung function as measured by **forced expiratory volume** is measurably reduced in people living in polluted areas but such data do not indicate which pollutant is

responsible and other factors may be equally important.

Experimental exposure of animals or human volunteers to individual pollutants shows toxic effects on pulmonary airways such as constriction and, hence, increased resistance, but **synergistic** effects occur between pollutants when they are present in mixtures. For example, the reaction between sulphur dioxide, water and ozone to give sulphuric acid is facilitated by the presence of hydrocarbons and particulates. Sulphur dioxide is an irritant but its lethal concentration is far greater than the amount normally encountered in air pollution. **Levels of sulphur dioxide** greater than **0.05 ppm** have been reputed to cause an increased incidence of respiratory illness and chronic exposure to levels above 0.2 ppm increased mortality. Exposure to levels of 1–5 ppm gives rise to acute discomfort. Smoke has a synergistic effect on sulphur dioxide toxicity so that the *combination* has a *greater* effect than either individual constituent.

Nitrogen dioxide and **ozone** are *more toxic* than sulphur dioxide and are deep lung irritants. Nitrogen oxides arise from car exhaust and other sources and cause respiratory symptoms at concentrations of 5–10 ppm. The levels of nitrogen oxides in Los Angeles average 0.7 ppm. Ozone causes damage to sensitive plants and affects humans suffering from asthma at levels of 50 ppb, yet in July 1976 concentrations of 260 ppb of ozone were measured in Britain and these levels were maintained for a week. The permitted level of ozone in factories is 80 ppb.

Carbon monoxide is another constituent of pollution, especially that derived from car exhausts. Although the chronic toxic effects of carbon monoxide are uncertain, the acute effects are well known (see Chapter 11). Carbon monoxide is very toxic, binding *avidly* to **haemoglobin** in competition with oxygen so as to reduce the ability of the blood to supply oxygen to the tissues. This will cause brain damage and death at high levels of blood saturation. It has been suggested that chronic exposure to carbon monoxide may cause heart damage resulting from tissue anoxia. Changes in blood pressure, pulse rate and cardiac output occur after 30 per cent saturation of blood with carbon monoxide, which is achieved at an ambient concentration of 75 ppm. The urban air concentration may be around 10–20 ppm resulting in about 4–8 per cent saturation. However, exposure levels as high as 100 ppm may be experienced in some circumstances such as by traffic policemen. These concentrations cause dizziness, headache and lassitude. Levels of 120 ppm for one hour or 30 ppm for eight hours are considered serious in the USA. Carbon monoxide is also present in **cigarette smoke** and heavy smoking may result in a level of more than 7 per cent carboxyhaemoglobin in the blood of the smoker. It is not clear whether exposure to carbon monoxide in the environment over the long term is a significant health hazard although it is believed to be an important factor in the cardiovascular effects of smoking. A positive correlation has been shown between carbon monoxide levels and myocardial infarction in Los Angeles but there were other confounding factors. Some individuals, however, such as those with anaemia who have low blood haemoglobin, are more sensitive to carbon monoxide than normal healthy people.

Pollution from power stations and especially car exhausts also contains **hydrocarbons** and these may be carcinogenic or have other toxic effects. The particulates present in smoke may become deposited in the lungs but this depends on the particle size as already described in Chapter 2. However, conclusive data on the effects of these pollutants on human health are not available. There are so many environmental factors which may adversely affect human health that attributing morbidity to a particular air pollutant is difficult.

Particulates

As well as airborne gases such as nitrogen oxides and substances such as lead, there are also particles present in the air we breathe. There is currently much concern about particular sized small particles, the so called **PM10**. These are particles which are less than 10 μm in diameter derived from cars and other vehicles. The particles vary in chemical composition but may simply be carbon emitted from car exhausts for example. There is increasing evidence that the levels of these in the air are connected to morbidity and mortality. The smallest of these particles can penetrate deep into the lungs and may therefore contribute to lung diseases. As well as a strong association between levels of particulates and deaths from respiratory diseases, there is also a correlation with hospital admissions and reports of symptoms of asthma (Bown, 1994).

Acid rain

In addition to having various effects on human health, pollutants may also be toxic to animals and plants in the environment and some of these effects can be demonstrated experimentally. One particular aspect of the environmental impact of pollutants currently of great concern is acid rain.

This term describes the **wet precipitation** of sulphuric and nitric acids and the **dry deposition** of sulphur dioxide, nitric acid and nitrogen oxides. It results from the burning of fossils fuels and certain industrial processes which produce sulphur dioxide and nitrogen oxides:

$$H_2O + SO_2 \xrightarrow{O_2;\ uv} H_2SO_4$$
$$\text{hydrocarbons}$$

$$NO_2 + H_2O \xrightarrow{H_2O;\ uv} HNO_3$$
$$\text{ozone}$$

These acids may be present in clouds and be removed during rain formation. This is known as **washout**. Alternatively they may be removed from the atmosphere by the falling rain. This is known as **rain-out**.

The effects of acid rain have been particularly noticeable in Scandinavia, partly as a result of the type of soil there. Sweden for example received about 472 000 tonnes of sulphur diox-ide in 1980 but only produced 240 000 tonnes, some of which would be deposited in other neighbouring countries, so Sweden suffered a net gain of 230 000 tonnes, despite having reduced its own production from 300 000 tonnes in 1978. Acid rain is clearly a world-wide pro-blem whereby the pollution is transported from one country to the next. Britain exports much of its pollution to Scandinavia and continental Europe (Figure 9.2) something which the power generating companies are now begin-ning to accept. Increased acidity has now been recognized in Britain itself, in Scotland and Snowdonia for example. The effects of acid rain depend on the type of deposition, the soil type and other factors. The *buffering* capacity of the soil is particularly important, but the thin soils found in parts of Scandinavia have poor

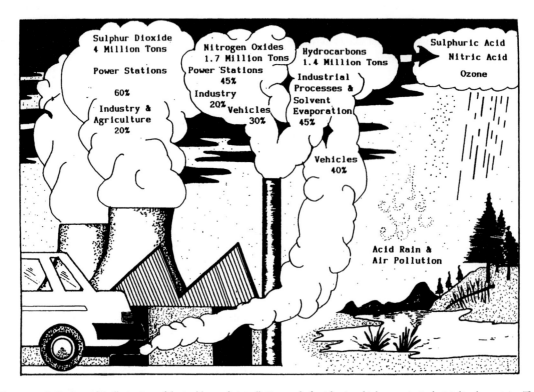

FIGURE 9.2 *A graphic illustration of the problems of air pollution and of acid rain which occur in industrialized countries. The figures give an indication of the situation in Great Britain at one time.*
Adapted from 'Why forests fear acid drops', The Sunday Times, *24 November 1985.*

buffering capacity and consequently the effects of the acidity are greater. The acidity in soil may also accumulate with time in some areas so that reducing the acid deposition will not have an immediate effect.

The sulphur and nitrogen oxides can cause rain, snow and mist to become acidic. Rain and snow mainly acidify the soil and ground water to a greater or lesser extent depending on the buffering capacity. The volume of rain or thaw water is also important for, if it is excessive, the water may overwhelm the natural buffers in the soil or saturate it. The water then runs straight into rivers and lakes with little contact with the bicarbonate and humus present in the soil which would buffer the acidity. Consequently, the rivers and lakes will become more acidic. Modern farming techniques, such as the use of **ammonium sulphate** fertilizers, may also exacerbate the increase in acidity. The actual acidity may cause certain organisms to die and will also upset the *balance* in the **ecosystem**. Water of *low* pH also *leaches* out metals such as **cadmium** and **lead** from the ground and causes **aluminium** salts to dissolve. These metals will damage plants if taken up by them and may also be toxic to animals. **Cadmium** is highly toxic to mammals, chronic exposure causing **kidney damage** and affecting bones in humans causing a **brittle bone syndrome**, which is known as **Itai-Itai** disease in Japan. **Aluminium** leached out of the soil and dissolved in acidic waters is believed to be one of the causes of the death of fish in Scandinavian lakes and rivers. One of the more vulnerable points is the reproductive cycle. How much damage wet deposition of acid causes to plants and especially trees is not yet clear. Dry deposition of sulphur dioxide, however, may damage leaves directly. There is serious damage to many types of **trees** in West Germany, and some estimate that 87 per cent of the firs are affected. This is now attributed to pollution. It may be due to a combination of factors and there is continuing discussion as to whether the major effect is acidification of the soil and

release of toxic metals or direct damage to the leaves or needles. Clearly air pollution contains a number of different compounds, but it seems that **ozone** is the constituent which is more likely to be directly toxic to trees rather than sulphur dioxide. Acidic ground water will not only leach out toxic metals which will be taken up by the tree but it will also leach out essential nutrients and so the soil will become deficient in them.

Acid rain may directly damage leaves on contact and will damage roots following seepage into soil. It will also wash out or displace essential elements from soil thereby leading to a deficiency in these nutrients. For example, magnesium lost from soil due to acidification is believed to be an important factor in the **dieback** of trees that has occurred in Germany. Increased acidity may also increase the mobility of metals in soil resulting in migration to lower levels in the soil and so out of reach of roots. However, the effects of acidification will vary due to the different buffering capacities of the soil in different geographical regions.

The pH of lakes and rivers may be affected directly by acid rain and indirectly by changes in the microorganisms and plants. Many species are adversely affected by a low pH. For example, in a number of rivers in Nova Scotia the pH fell from 5.7 to 4.9 over the period 1954–73. During this period there has also been a fall in the number of Atlantic salmon. The balance between particular species of animal or plant will also alter as a result of acidification, some being lost and others thriving. Overall, however, there is a reduction in diversity.

Most scientists involved now agree that all of the constituents of pollution, from both power stations and cars, should be reduced as much as possible even though it is not yet clear which ones are the most important. However, some scientists and some Governments have argued that reducing sulphur dioxide, for example, may have little effect if the important determining factor is the level of ozone or hydrocarbons which catalyze the conversion of sulphur dioxide and nitrogen oxides to sulphuric acid and nitric acid respectively. It is possible, however, to remove some of the sulphur dioxide from the smoke derived from fossil fuels before, during and after burning. Similarly, the output of carbon monoxide, nitrogen oxides and hydrocarbons from car exhausts can be reduced with **catalytic converters**. These are already in use in some countries and in the USA emissions of carbon monoxide and hydrocarbons from new cars have fallen by 90 per cent and nitrogen oxides by 75 per cent between 1970 and 1983. Two of these pollutants, nitrogen oxides and hydrocarbons, are involved in the production of ozone in the atmosphere and nitrogen oxides also contribute to acid rain as already described. In the view of British scientists at Harwell, *reducing* **hydrocarbons** in car exhausts is the best way to reduce atmospheric ozone. It should be noted, however, that some ozone in the atmosphere is necessary and that if the atmospheric level drops too low then more ultraviolet light reaches the surface of the earth, possibly leading to an increase in skin cancer. The **chlorofluorocarbons** used as aerosol propellants are believed to be one cause of a *reduction* in atmospheric ozone.

Perhaps when the real extent and economic consequences of the damage due to these pollutants such as to buildings and metal structures as well as to trees and humans become known, governments will enact legislation to cause a major reduction in output pollutants from all sources.

Lead pollution

Another major environmental pollutant is lead, known to be a poisonous compound for centuries. Its toxicity was certainly recognized by 300

BC as a case of **lead poisoning** was described by **Hippocrates** around that time. For centuries workers involved in lead mining and smelting have been occupationally exposed. Lead poisoning may even have contributed to the decline of the Roman Empire as high lead levels have been detected in Roman skeletons from that period. Lead pollution arises mainly from car exhausts but industrial processes, batteries, minerals and **lead arsenate** insecticide also contribute to lead in the environment. The use of cooking vessels with lead glaze or made of lead may have been another source in earlier times. Industrial poisoning became common in the Industrial Revolution, with a *thousand cases a year* in the UK alone at the end of the nineteenth century. However, a relatively recent study by the EEC in Glasgow showed that 10 per cent of babies had > 0.3 μg ml^{-1} of lead in their blood indicating that there is still cause for concern. Lead is taken in from food, via the lungs and from water and although the amount found in food may be greater than that in air, the absorption is greater from the lungs than from the gut. Children are more susceptible than adults as they *absorb greater amounts* from the gastrointestinal tract.

It has been estimated that 98 per cent of the airborne lead in the UK is derived from leaded petrol and levels of lead in the air correlate with the amount of traffic. The lead in car exhausts is derived from **tetraethyl lead**, an anti-knock compound added to petrol which is converted to lead in the engine. Certain individuals, such as traffic policemen, may have higher blood lead levels than the average member of the urban population because they have greater exposure to car exhausts. **Cigarette smoke** is also a source of inhaled lead.

At the beginning of the twentieth century large-scale poisoning of children with lead became known, especially of those living in poor housing in slum areas of the USA. The source of this lead was mainly from paint containing relatively large amounts of lead. The paint was taken in by children through contamination of food or fingers or perhaps by experimental tasting of flakes of paint. In children, the most serious effect of lead poisoning is **encephalopathy** with mental retardation, and seizures and cerebral palsy may be lifelong effects. The nervous system is a clear target for lead and is particularly susceptible in young children. A cause for concern is whether even a single episode of poisoning is sufficient to cause permanent damage in children.

After absorption, lead enters the blood where 97 per cent is taken up by the **red blood cell**. The half-life of lead in the red blood cell is 2–3 weeks. Some redistribution of the lead to liver and kidney occurs and then excretion into the **bile** or deposition in **bone** takes place. In bone the lead eventually becomes incorporated into the hydroxyapatite crystal. Due to this deposition in bone and teeth it is possible to estimate past exposure to lead by X-ray analysis. It is also possible to detect lead poisoning and exposure from urine and blood analysis as the amount in blood represents the current exposure.

The 'normal' blood levels in the USA have been reported as between **0.15–0.7 μg ml^{-1}** with an average at 0.3 μg ml^{-1}. The threshold for **toxicity** is **0.8 μg ml^{-1}**, and encephalopathy occurs at 1–2 μg ml^{-1}. However, biochemical effects can be seen at lower levels: lead interferes with **haem** and **porphyrin synthesis** and its effects on the enzymes of this pathway can be demonstrated (Figure 9.3); myoglobin synthesis and cytochrome P450 may also be affected. The results of the effects on porphyrin synthesis are a reduction in haemoglobin level, the appearance of **coproporphyrin** and **aminolaevulinic acid** (ALA) in the urine. Free **erythrocyte protoporphyrin** is increased and **aminolaevulinic acid dehydrase** (ALAD) is inhibited. Inhibition of ALAD is the most sensitive measure of exposure and in human sub-

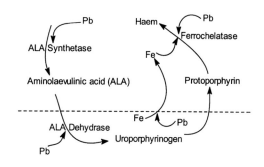

Mitochondrion

Cytosol

FIGURE 9.3 *The synthesis of haem in the mammalian erythrocyte. The points at which lead (Pb) interferes with this synthetic pathway are shown.*

jects there is a correlation between blood lead and the degree of inhibition of the enzyme. At blood levels of 0.4 μg ml^{-1} ALAD is inhibited to the extent of 50 per cent. At levels of 0.6–0.8 μg ml^{-1} there is a greater effect and mild symptoms; at levels of 0.8–1.0 μg ml^{-1} there are more definite clinical signs; at levels of 1–2 μg ml^{-1} encephalopathy occurs. The symptoms are non-specific **colic** and **abdominal pain, lassitude** and **constipation. Anaemia** occurs later and CNS effects occur after prolonged exposure. The blood lead level rises and ALAD falls within a few days of exposure. The ALA and coproporphyrin in urine increase after two weeks.

Lead interferes at several steps in haem synthesis: with the enzymes **ferrochelatase, aminolaevulinate synthetase** (ALAS) and **aminolaevulinate dehydrase** (ALAD), and with the **uptake of iron** into the mitochondrion. Increased excretion of ALA in the urine is one marker for lead exposure. In 1970 10 per cent of all children in New York and Chicago had blood levels of 0.6 μg ml^{-1}. Many of these children lived in good housing. As with carbon monoxide exposure anaemic individuals who have a low haemoglobin level and reduced red blood cell count may be more at risk as their lead carrying capacity is lower and the amount of haemoglobin is already low. Anaemia may result from lead exposure partly as a result of inhibition of haemoglobin synthesis and partly by causing the destruction of red blood cells.

Measurement of the inhibition of ALAD is too sensitive a measure of lead exposure, whereas the presence of haemoglobin and coproporphyrin in urine occurs after severe damage. The detection of ALA in urine is the most useful method for determination of lead poisoning.

As well as affecting the CNS and haem synthesis, in children lead also causes **skeletal changes** following chronic exposure. Bands at the growing ends of long bones can be detected and bone shape may also be affected. Chronic exposure may also be detected by a lead line on the gums. Acute exposure to lead may also cause **kidney damage**, while chronic exposure may lead to interstitial **nephritis**. This may be the cause of the nephritis associated with drinking moonshine whisky as the stills used sometimes contained lead piping or lead solder.

Whether lead in the atmosphere in cities poses a real threat to the mental health of children is currently disputed. Barltrop does not believe that the data shows there is a clear relationship between the body lead burden and IQ decreases in children but it may be difficult to prove such a relationship. In the UK there have been three reports on this: by the DHSS, by a Royal Commission and by the Medical Research Council; all have concluded that many of the studies on this aspect of lead poisoning were inadequate. Studies are under way to look at blood lead levels of 0.4–0.8 μg ml^{-1} in relation to the function of the central and peripheral nervous system. It has been suggested that subclinical disease of the central and peripheral nervous system and kidney may follow long-term exposure at levels to which the general population are exposed in the urban environment. This is very difficult,

however, if not impossible to prove in the human population.

So far we have been considering inorganic lead, yet **organic lead** is probably *more toxic* as it is lipid-soluble and therefore well absorbed. For example, triethyl lead, which results from combustion of petrol containing tetraethyl lead, is readily taken up through skin and into the brain and will cause **encephalopathy**. This has been the cause of toxic effects in workers exposed in industry where the tetraethyl lead is manufactured. The effects occur rapidly and the symptoms are **delusions**, **hallucinations** and **ataxia**.

How much of a hazard the levels of lead in our air, food and water pose to the health of children and adults is currently unclear. However, it is probable that we could remove much of that pollution and the hazard by removing lead from petrol without any major effect on petrol prices or car performance. Lead is known from both animal and human studies to be highly toxic and the levels to which many of us are exposed can be shown to have effects on biochemical pathways. It is surely only prudent to reduce the exposure to this toxic metal as much as possible by reducing its use and release into the environment.

Water pollution

Water in rivers, lakes and the sea may be polluted directly by the discharge of effluent from factories and industrial processes, and of domestic waste. Water may become polluted also by substances on the land such as pesticides and fertilizers applied to crops and washed by rain into rivers and lakes and eventually into the sea. The rain can also directly accumulate substances from the atmosphere. Industrial companies may dump toxic waste into underground storage tanks and leakage of these has been known to lead to contamination of the water table. The domestic water supply in such areas then becomes contaminated.

Some water pollutants, such as **fertilizers** from agricultural run-off, **sewage** and **organic waste products** from the food industry lead to overgrowth of **algae** and other aquatic plants which eventually choke the local environment and use up the available **nutrients**. The algae then die, and decay with the help of **aerobic bacteria** which use up the oxygen in the water. This is followed by the appearance of **anaerobic bacteria** which continue to feed from the decaying plant matter at the bottom of the lake or river. These bacteria produce toxic compounds which, along with the lack of oxygen, cause the water to become stagnant and so other aquatic organisms such as fish die. This process is known as **eutrophication**.

Humans, other animals and plants may become exposed to toxic pollutants in water either by drinking that water, living in it or eating other organisms which have become contaminated by it. Although in Western nations drinking water is normally highly purified, this may not be the case in less developed countries. However some toxic substances, such as heavy metals, are not necessarily removed by the normal water-treatment procedures.

Water pollutants may affect organisms within the environment in different ways. High concentrations of a toxic compound may kill most or all of the organisms within a particular area where the concentration is sufficiently high. However, this area may become repopulated in time from another area. A more insidious pollutant may damage the reproductive cycle of certain organisms in some way. Fish eggs are very susceptible to toxic compounds at low levels for example and this may lead to a decline in the fish population.

Another way in which a pollutant can interact with the environment is by entering **food chains** (see below), without causing damage to the lower organisms in the chain, but possibly killing the predators at the top of the chain or interfering with their reproductive cycle. Persistent compounds such as **methyl mercury** and **DDT** enter food chains and act in this way.

The pollutant may not however remain the same once it is in the environment as it may be altered by chemical or biochemical processes. Consequently, two important aspects of environmental pollution are the involvement of food chains and the alteration of the compound by the environment itself.

Arsenic

This element is widely distributed in the Earth's crust and is associated with ores used for zinc, copper, gold and lead extraction. The mining of these ores is therefore an important source of exposure. Arsenic is also used in pesticides. Although seafood may be contaminated with arsenic this may be in the organic form which is less toxic than the inorganic form. Also water from ground water wells and hot springs may be naturally contaminated with arsenic.

Ground water is a significant source of arsenic poisoning and in some parts of the world levels may be especially high. For example in Taiwan levels as high as 1.8 mg^{-1} have been recorded. Significant contamination of water also occurs in Bangladesh and Argentina. In Bangladesh there has been a particular problem of wells contaminated with arsenic from ground water being used to replace wells contaminated with bacteria and this arsenic contamination has led to widescale disease. In this and other countries with high levels of contamination, chronic exposure to arsenic causes hyperpigmentation of the skin, keratosis and cancer. It may also cause a peripheral vascular disorder known as **black-foot disease** which has been reported in Taiwan. In both Taiwan and Argentina, **skin cancer** has been associated with exposure to high levels.

Food chains

For a terrestrial animal the most likely route of exposure to a toxic compound such as a pollutant is via its **food**. The food chain is one method by which animals and man become exposed to persistent pollutants. Substances may however be persistent in one environment or species but not in another, depending on the particular characteristics of the system. The food chain can involve water-borne pollutants and also soil and airborne pollutants. There are two main types of food chain; **grazing** and **detritivore**. A grazing food chain is a sequence in which one organism, such as a plant, is eaten by another such as a herbivore which is in turn eaten by a carnivore and so on (Table 8.3). A detritivore food chain involves the decay of organisms after death. The organisms involved tend to be small and there is no increase in size between the lower and higher trophic levels. Both types of food chain can be involved in environmental toxicology as can other types of feeding relationships. The overall system may be termed a food web.

The amounts of a pollutant in species at each trophic level (Table 8.3) may be measured and compared to give a concentration factor. However, these must be interpreted with caution. For example, the mode of **sampling** a population may have inherent **bias**. Ideally sampling should be random, but it may not always be so. If animal carcasses are sampled the levels of a particular pollutant may vary widely depending on the cause of death.

Indeed the concentration of pollutant in live animals may be at least as important as the concentration in those dying of unknown cause. This is because the pollutant may have subtle population effects, such as on breeding behaviour or the production of eggs, which will affect the whole population. Another important point is that the mere presence of a chemical in the environment does not necessarily mean there has been significant pollution and similarly the presence of a chemical in an organism does not necessarily mean that it is causing toxic effects. Our *ability* to measure toxic compounds at minute levels should not blind us to the necessity for a reasonable assessment and *interpretation* of those data. Unlike controlled laboratory experiments, environmental exposure may often be intermittent and pollutants do not always reach a steady state but can fluctuate wildly. As already mentioned, persistence of a chemical can vary between species or ecosystems. For example, it has been reported that small mammals may have a low level of organochlorine insecticides whilst birds feeding on them may have very high and possibly lethal levels. This may be due to differences in the metabolism of the pollutant by the two species.

Thus, the mammal might eliminate the substance relatively rapidly whereas the bird may not and so it will *accumulate*. Again sampling can be an important factor in studying this problem as predators may take prey from a wide area in which there are great variations in exposure. It is clear that environmental toxicology deals with complex systems in which prediction is sometimes very difficult.

Although the effects of pollutants on individual human beings may be perceived by man as the most important, ecologically and biologically an effect on the population may be more important. Consequently, a pollutant which reduces or stops reproduction of the species at some stage is more important than a pollutant which is more acutely toxic but only causes the death of the older, more susceptible members of that species. The latter would be more obviously distressing but would have *less effect* on the population if the victims were past significant reproductive capacity. The toxic compound would be just one more cause of death. Indeed not all individuals in a population reproduce and so there may be less effect than might be expected for a toxic pollutant which leads to the death of only some members of that population.

An example which illustrates this effect on the reproductive cycle and the problems of persistent pesticides in food chains is the effect of **organochlorine** insecticides on **eggshells** in predatory birds, as mentioned in Chapter 8. The predatory bird is at the top of a food chain and hence may have the highest concentration of pollutant. The **peregrine falcon** population in Britain declined precipitately between 1955 and 1962. At the same time the frequency of egg breakage increased because of a decrease in eggshell thickness. There is a linear relationship between eggshell strength and the thickness index. Peregrine falcon eggs studied during the period 1970–1974 had a lower thickness index and strength than those studied between 1850 and 1942. **DDE**, a metabolite of DDT is believed to be one cause of this decreased thickness. Direct toxicity of **dieldrin** to falcons has been suggested as another cause of the decline in population. Areas such as the north of Scotland had a higher eggshell thickness index and lower levels of DDE than eggs from more southern areas of the UK. Similarly data from the USA for kestrels showed a correlation between eggshell thickness and DDE concentration (Figure 8.2).

Pollutants which contaminate water may either dissolve in it if they are ionized/water-soluble substances or are miscible. Alternatively if they are hydrophobic they may form a suspension or aggregate and remain undispersed in the same manner as the familiar oil slick. Although water-soluble substances may reach a sufficient concentration to be toxic to aquatic organisms and to man, unless they are in an enclosed system they will tend to disperse eventually. Such compounds are not likely to accumulate in organisms. Hydrophobic substances however behave differently. Substances which are not polar and are soluble in lipid rather than water are well absorbed by living organisms especially by aquatic organisms which pass water over gills to extract oxygen and to filter water in search of food. Consequently, small organisms such as *Daphnia* and **zooplankton** become contaminated with lipophilic pollutants such as DDT. These small organisms are then eaten by other, larger organisms such as small fish and the contaminant enters the fatty tissue of this larger organism. However, if the small organisms are ingested in large numbers and the compound is not readily excreted, the concentration of the substance in the larger organism increases. This process is repeated with ever larger and larger organisms until the ultimate predator, at the top of the food chain may accumulate sufficient of the substance to suffer toxic effects (Table 8.3; Figure 9.4). Food chains may occur in aquatic environments with water pollutants, or in terrestrial organisms with airborne, soil, water or food borne pollutants, or a combination of these. The important aspect of any food chain, therefore, is the scope for **biomagnification** of the substance as it moves up through the chain. Furthermore the compound may be non-toxic at the low levels encountered by the organisms at the bottom of the chain which therefore survive and contaminate the predators further up the chain.

The most important characteristics of a substance which enters a food chain are its **lipid solubility** and its **metabolic stability** in biological systems. These determine the extent to which the compound is taken up by the organism and its ability to localize in fat tissue and remain there until the organism is ingested by a predator. Hydrophilic compounds, which are polar and ionized, may be taken up by organisms but will tend to be readily excreted. Lipophilic pollutants which are absorbed and then *rapidly metabolized* to *polar metabolites* similarly tend to be *readily excreted* and hence will not persist in the organism or be transferred to the predator.

This is another example of the importance of **physico-chemical characteristics** in toxicology.

Although some environmental pollutants are not lipophilic initially they may be *metabolized* by micro-organisms, plants or higher animals to lipophilic metabolites which are more persistent. DDT is an example of this; its metabolite DDE is more lipophilic and much more persistent (Figure 8.1 and Table 8.2). Another is inorganic mercury (see page 138).

Endocrine disruptors

'Endocrine disruptors are exogenous substances which cause adverse health effects in an intact organism or its progeny subsequent to changes in endocrine function'.

Over recent years a number of coincident observations have led scientists to the conclusion that chemical substances in the environment may be interfering with the endocrine systems of humans and various animals. These so-called endocrine disruptors may be responsible for a range of dysfunctions in the reproductive systems of humans and a variety of animals in the wild. The wildlife effects are well documented and some can be reproduced experimentally. The human effects are more

difficult to definitively associate with environmental chemicals and some effects are controversial.

However, there is considerable interest in the area which is potentially of great importance.

It is widely accepted that chemicals that are capable of causing endocrine disruption have been released into the environment. These chemicals may act as **oestrogen mimics**, as **anti-oestrogens** or as **anti-androgens**. The end result is a change in the hormone balance which may result in a variety of physiological and pathological effects. The debate, however, is whether the concentrations of these chemicals is sufficient to cause all of the effects undoubtedly observed in animals and the effects suspected as being related in humans.

There is a variety of chemicals believed to be responsible, most of which are man-made but some natural chemicals from plants or fungi are included as well. The chemicals include **organochlorine insecticides** (e.g. DDT) and industrial chemicals such as **polychlorinated biphenyls (PCB's)** and **alkylphenols** and drugs such as used in the **contraceptive pill** and **diethylstilboestrol** and synthetic oestrogens which are excreted into the urine and hence appear in rivers via sewage. Natural products include the fungal product **zearalenone** and the plant product **genistein**. Some of the chemicals are lipophilic and persistent, undergoing bioaccumulation and biomagnification in the environment.

WILDLIFE EFFECTS

The evidence for, and examples of, endocrine disruption in wildlife comes from many parts of the world over a number of years and in a variety of animal species ranging from molluscs to alligators. One of the first observations was of changes in fish in rivers in the UK and in the USA. It was noticed that some fish (roach and rainbow trout in the UK and winter flounder in the USA) in rivers polluted with sewage outfall or industrial effluent were showing **hermaphroditism**. The incidence of intersex was as much as 100% of the fish in the river Aire in the UK. Male fish were also found to be producing vitellogenin, a protein which female fish produce in response to oestrogen. This response could be reproduced experimentally when fish were exposed to sewage. **Vitellogenin** is therefore a biomarker of response for the effect of certain chemical substances on fish.

Some of the specific substances that cause male fish to produce vitellogenin, such as the alkylphenols, **octylphenol** and **nonylphenol**, have now been identified. These compounds also decrease testicular growth in fish and bind to the oestrogen receptor. However, although nonylphenol is potent, it is still very much less potent than natural oestrogen. However, it has also been shown that the synthetic oestrogen, **ethynyloestradiol**, will, at concentrations found in the effluent from sewage treatment works, cause male fish to produce vitellogenin and will retard testes growth.

Plant steroids have also been suspected of causing masculinization in female fish. Such compounds are found in the effluent from paper mills.

A well described and studied effect of an environmental pollutant on the reproductive system of aquatic organisms is the effect of tributyl tin on molluscs. **Tributyl tin oxide (TBTO)** is used as a biocide in wood preservatives and in paints used for the undersides of small boats to stop fouling by algae and barnacles. The tributyl tin concentration in crowded harbours and marinas may be sufficient to cause effects on molluscs such as the **dog whelk**. Molluscs appear to be especially sensitive to the effects of tributyl tin and concentrations of less than 1 ng per litre will produce adverse effects. The results of the exposure are imposex, in which females become masculinized with the growth of a penis. This effect has been observed in many parts of the world with a large number of different species of marine snails and also have been reproduced in the laboratory.

The mechanism may involve inhibition of **aromatase**, an enzyme involved in the metabolism of sex hormones. Tributyl tin also has other toxic effects in mammals causing damage to the thymus. This leads to depletion of lymphocytes and so adversely affects the immune system. However, this occurs at concentrations several orders of magnitude higher than those which cause imposex in molluscs.

However, the most celebrated example of endocrine disruption is that caused by organochlorine compounds in alligators in Florida. It was reported that the population of alligators in **Lake Apopka** in Northern Florida was declining. This seemed to be due to poor reproductive success. The male animals had small phalli, poorly organized testes and low testosterone levels. In contrast the females had high oestrogen levels but abnormal ovarian morphology. The mechanism was suggested as being due to an effect of the pollutants on the metabolism of steroid sex hormones. There was clearly a high level of pollution by organochlorine compounds such as the DDT breakdown product DDE. This compound has been shown experimentally to have reproductive and hormonal effects in alligators.

HUMAN EFFECTS

There are a number of effects on the human reproductive system that have been observed and documented. Although some are contentious, some are clearly established.

There has been an undeniable increase in **testicular cancer** and **breast cancer** over the period since 1945 particularly in certain countries. It is also suggested by some, but not all data, that **sperm counts** and **sperm quality** in men has declined over the same period. This seems particularly apparent in some Scandinavian countries but is not supported by data from some other countries. There may also be an increase in other disorders of the male reproductive system such as **cryptorchidism** and **hypospadia**.

In contrast to the effects observed and reproduced in animals, the effects on human reproductive function and the organs involved, while documented, have not been clearly associated with exposure to particular chemicals. The notable exception to this is diethylstilboestrol which was used therapeutically in the 1950s to prevent miscarriages in women until its use was stopped in the early 1970s. This synthetic oestrogen was found to cause problems in the reproductive systems of the male and female offspring of women who had received the drug. These findings lend credence to the hypothesis that oestrogenic compounds could be responsible for some at least of the observed effects. This substance has also been administered to animals in which similar effects have been recorded.

In a significant proportion of girls born to mothers who had been prescribed diethylstilboestrol there was dysfunction of the reproductive organs, disruption of the menstrual cycle and abnormal pregnancies. In a small number, adenocarcinoma of the vagina developed when the girls reached puberty. Male offspring showed increased incidence of cryptorchidism and microphallus. There was some evidence of decreased sperm count and motility. These effects and also testicular cancer have been reproduced in experimental animals. As diethylstilboestrol does not bind to sex hormone binding globulin it is able to enter cells freely and therefore has a greater effect than an equivalent blood concentration of endogenous oestrogens.

Diethylstilboestrol was also used as a growth promoter in cattle and so humans may also have been exposed to residues in meat. Human exposure to the synthetic oestrogens used in the contraceptive pill may occur via the drinking water. Ethynyloestradiol has been detected in drinking water in the UK but the data have been questioned. Metabolites of such compounds as well as natural oestrogens will be excreted into urine and thence may find their way into drinking water or contaminate crops, via the sewage system. This could be more of a problem in times of drought when concentrations may be higher.

Although DDT has been implicated as a possible xenoestrogen, it does not interact significantly with the oestrogen receptor and nor does its persistent metabolite p,p'-DDE. However, **p,p'-DDE** *does* interact with the **androgen receptor** and therefore could conceivably be an anti-androgen and this may warrant further study. Studies have measured DDE in breast adipose tissue in an attempt to correlate the levels with the incidence of breast cancer but the results have been equivocal. It has been suggested that there may be a slight association with only the hormone responsive type of breast cancer. However, it should be noted that the current exposure of the human population to DDT is relatively low and continually decreasing. Furthermore, studies of humans exposed to very much higher levels of DDT when it was first introduced, especially in those manufacturing and using the compound have revealed little toxicity. The organochlorine compound **chlordecone**, however, has been shown to have oestrogen-like activity in humans. Male workers exposed to high levels during its manufacture were found to have changes in the reproductive system including abnormal sperm with decreased motility and low sperm counts. Although some **polychlori-**

nated **biphenyls (PCBs)** possess weak oestrogenic activity, others are anti-oestrogenic.
Similarly, **dioxin (TCDD)** shows significant
anti-oestrogenic activity. In both cases the
activity seems to be correlated with the binding
to the **Ah receptor**. Dioxin has a number of
effects on the male and female reproductive
systems of mammals, for example having
adverse effects on spermatogenesis, sexual
behaviour and reproductive capability. Effects
on the reproductive system have been shown
at doses as low as 0.001 μg/kgbw/day in rats
and monkeys. After one human exposure situation, **Seveso** in Italy in 1976, studies in fact
revealed a *decreased* incidence of breast
cancer.

Alkylphenols, such as octylphenol, do show
oestrogenic activity which appears to be
mediated via the oestrogen receptor.
However, the activity is three orders of magnitude less than oestradiol and the likelihood of
effects on humans is probably low.

Finally, it should be noted that there are
many naturally occurring oestrogens which,
although many times less potent than oestradiol, may have far greater potency than some
of the man-made chemicals often mentioned.
Thus, the plant products **isoflavone**, **coume-
stans** and **lignane** and the fungal product **zeal-
arone**, all bind to the oestrogen receptor. Other
plant-derived products such as **indole-3-carbi-
nol** found in vegetables, have anti-oestrogenic
activity.

It is clear that there is human exposure to a
wide variety of compounds in the environment
which have some oestrogenic activity (xenoestrogens) and some anti-oestrogenic activity.
Whether many of these individually at the likely
exposure concentrations pose a threat to
human reproductive health is still unclear.
However, our environment contains many
such compounds and so combinations of
weakly oestrogenic compounds may show
synergy so that significant oestrogenic activity

results. This is an area currently receiving considerable attention.

Xenoestrogens may act through other pathways than via the oestrogen receptor. For
example, they can interact with other receptors such as the Ah receptor or the growth
factor receptor. Indeed, there seems to be
an association between binding to the Ah
receptor and anti-oestrogenic activity.
Alternatively, some xenoestrogens may act
by altering oestrogen metabolism. For example, 17β-oestradiol is metabolized to both 2-
hydroxyoestrone and 16α-hydroxyoestrone. 2-
Hydroxyoestrone has low activity and low
genotoxicity whereas **16α-hydroxyoestrone is
genotoxic** and is a **potent oestrogen**. In
breast cancer patients it has been found that
levels of 16α-hydroxyoestrone are higher than
in control patients and that the ratio of 16α-
hydroxy to 2-hydroxy oestrone is associated
with breast cancer. Some polycyclic aromatic
hydrocarbons for instance inhibit the formation of 2-hydroxyoestrone and so divert the
metabolism of oestradiol towards the more
potent 16α-hydroxyoestrone.

Another, alternative mechanism for affecting
the reproductive system, is if a chemical pos-
sesses anti-androgenic activity.

Mercury and methylmercury

Mercury is 'the hottest, the coldest, a true
healer, a wicked murderer, a precious medicine, and a deadly poison, a friend that can
flatter and lie.' (Woodall, J. (1639) *The
Surgeon' Mate or Military & Domestic Surgery.*
London, p. 256, quoted from *Casarett and
Doull's Toxicology.)*

Like lead, mercury is a highly toxic metal the
toxic properties of which have been known
about for centuries. The phrase 'Mad as a

Hatter' has its origins in the effects on exposed workers of the mercury salts used to cure felt for hats. Mercury and its salts have been used in many ways for centuries. In the Middle Ages it was used to treat syphilis.

Mercury exists in three chemical forms: elemental, inorganic and organic. All three forms are toxic in different ways. **Elemental mercury (Hg^0)**, often used in scientific instruments, is absorbed as the vapour and is highly toxic. Mercury readily vaporizes even at room temperature and exposure to it can lead to damage to the **central nervous system**. **Inorganic mercury (Hg^+ and Hg^{2+})**, in mercury salts, is not readily absorbed but when it does gain access to the body, it causes mainly **kidney damage**. **Organic mercury** compounds (R-Hg^+) are readily absorbed by living organisms and, therefore, are more hazardous than inorganic mercury. As with elemental mercury, the target is the **brain** and **nervous system**.

The different forms of mercury may act by basically similar mechanisms of action involving the reaction of the metal or its ions with **sulphydryl groups**. These sulphydryl groups may be part of a protein, such as an enzyme, and hence mercury is a potent inhibitor of enzymes in which the SH group is important. The differences in the toxicity of the three forms of mercury are due to differences in distribution. Elemental mercury is readily taken up from the lungs and is oxidized in red blood cells to Hg^{2+}. Hg^0 is also readily taken up into the brain and the foetus and is also metabolized to Hg^{2+} in these tissues. The mercury is then trapped in these sites by virtue of being ionized. Consequently elemental mercury causes mainly neurological damage. Inorganic mercury cannot cross the blood-brain barrier, but reaches the kidney and it is this organ particularly that is damaged. Organic mercury is sufficiently lipid-soluble to distribute to the central nervous system where it also is oxidized to Hg^{2+}, and causes mainly neurological damage. So,

although all three forms of mercury are probably toxic as a result of binding to sulphydryl groups in proteins, the *differences in distribution* lead to differences in the type of toxicity. This is another illustration of the importance of distribution in the toxicity of foreign compounds.

Exposure to mercury used to be mainly an occupational hazard rather than an environmental one, but more recently mercury has also become an environmental pollutant. This has occurred through the use of **organomercury fungicides** and through the industrial use of mercury in the manufacture of plastics, paper and batteries with the resultant discharge of the contaminated effluents into lakes and rivers. High levels have been detected, as in water near a battery plant in Michigan, where levels of 1000 ppm were found when the permissible level was 5 ppb. Mercury has also been detected in air, presumably arising from industrial processes.

Dumping of the inorganic form of the metal used to be tolerated because it was thought that this form was relatively innocuous and easily dispersed.

The use of mercury-containing fungicides has led to water contamination via run-off from fields. Other sources of environmental mercury are wood pulp plants and chloroalkali plants. These and possibly other sources were presumably responsible for the contamination of freshwater fish by high levels of mercury detected by Swedish scientists. As with other lipid-soluble substances in the environment, bioconcentration in the food chain also occurs.

Mercury dumping is now controlled and organomercury fungicides are being phased out.

A tragic and now infamous event, which occurred in Japan in the 1950s, highlighted the dangers of inorganic mercury as a water pollutant. In 1956 a new factory on the shores of **Minamata Bay** in Japan began producing vinyl chloride and acetaldehyde. Mercuric chloride was used as a catalyst, and after use was discharged into the bay with the rest of the effluent from the factory. Within a year a new illness had appeared among the local fishermen and their families which became known as **Minamata Disease**. Their pet cats also suffered similar symptoms. It was eventually recognized that the disease was due to contaminated seafood and mercury was suspected in 1959. **Methylmercury** was detected in seafood in 1960 and in sediments derived from the factory in 1961. The methylmercury was being taken up by the seafood which was eaten by the local population. A food chain was involved with the organic mercury being concentrated by the aquatic organisms because, unlike inorganic mercury it is lipid-soluble. It became apparent that the inorganic mercury that discharged into rivers, lakes or the sea was not inert but could be *biomethylated* to methylmercury by micro-organisms (Figure 9.4). This occurred especially under *anaerobic* conditions, such as in the effluent sludge which collected at the bottom of Minamata Bay. This highlighted the fact that inorganic mercury dumped into rivers and lakes is by no means innocuous and is not necessarily dispersed.

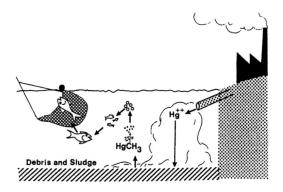

FIGURE 9.4 *The way in which inorganic mercury in effluent was taken up into the food chain and led to the poisoning of several hundred local inhabitants in Minamata Bay in Japan. The inorganic mercury was methylated by micro-organisms in the anaerobic sludge lying at the bottom of the bay and so became more soluble in fatty tissue and was easily taken up into living organisms.*

The contamination at Minamata led to 700 cases of poisoning and over 70 deaths. Diversion of effluent by the factory eliminated the disease. Mass poisonings have also occurred in various parts of the world as a result of the use of organomercury compounds as fungicides to treat seed grain. The treated grain should not be used as food but if it is used to feed livestock, the meat becomes contaminated. One such large-scale poisoning incident occurred in Iraq in 1971–1972 when alkylmercury fungicides were used to treat cereal grain. This involved 6000 people and resulted in 500 deaths.

In another incident in 1969, a New Mexico family fed treated grain to pigs, and then ate the pigs. Three of the ten children exposed experienced behavioural abnormalities and other neurological disorders. A child exposed *in utero* was born with brain damage and the urinary level of mercury was found to be *15 times* that of the mother.

The symptoms of methylmercury poisoning reflect the entry of the compound into the central nervous system, beginning with memory loss, paresthesias, ataxia, narrowing of the visual field, and progressing to loss of muscle co-ordination and emotional instability and eventually **cerebral palsy**. The latter was the most distressing effect seen at Minamata. Children and new born infants seemed to be most severely affected and those exposed *in utero* were born with severe cerebral palsy even when the mothers were symptom-free, a classic characteristic of a **teratogen**. Methylmercury is able to cross the placenta and may consequently *concentrate* in the fat tissue and brain of the embryo and foetus. In addition, foetal red blood cells concentrate methylmercury 30 per cent more than the adult red blood cells. The damage caused by methylmercury is permanent.

The methylmercury that enters the brain is demethylated and the inorganic mercury released can then bind to the **sulphydryl groups** of enzymes and inactivate them. Methylmercury has a *long half-life* in the body, approximately 70 days. It is localized particularly in the liver and brain, with 10–20 per cent of the body burden of mercury in the brain. It is possible to calculate from this and the known toxic concentration that the **allowable daily intake** with a safety factor of 10 would be 0.1 mg day^{-1} This would correspond to eating 200 g of fish with a mercury level of 0.5 ppm, but fish in Lake Michigan and in the sea off the coast of Sweden have been found to contain as much as *ten times* more mercury than this in some cases.

Like humans, birds and other animals may ingest mercury. For example, studies of the Crested Grebe show that tissue mercury levels have been steadily increasing since about 1870 (Figure 9.5).

Substances, such as pesticides and other chemicals, which may contaminate the environment have to be tested for toxicity in a variety of species including fish, *Daphnia*, honey bees and earthworms. Also, **ecotoxicity testing** requires determination of the **biochemical and chemical oxygen demand**, abbreviated BOD and COD respectively. The **BOD** indicates the ability of micro-organisms to metabolize an organic substance. The **COD** is the amount of oxygen required to oxidize the substance chemically. The ratio of the COD and BOD is an indication of the *biodegradability* of the substance. There are a number of other tests which will give an indication of the persistence of the compound in the environment such as determination of abiotic degradation. Details of these can be found in the documents issued by such governmental organizations as the Environmental Protection Agency (EPA) in the USA and the Health and Safety Executive (HSE) in Britain.

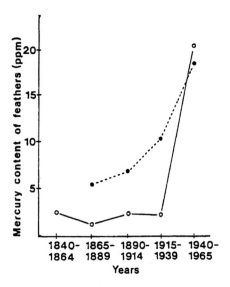

FIGURE 9.5 *The increase in mercury levels detected in two species of birds, Crested Grebe (●) and Goshawk (○), over a 100-year period. The mercury content was determined in feathers from museum specimens of Swedish birds. Data from Wallace et al. (1971) Mercury in the Environment: The Human Element, ORNL-NSF Environmental Program, Oak Ridge National Laboratory, Figure 4.*

Summary and learning objectives

Exposure (via skin contact, oral intake, breathing) of biological systems to chemicals may occur through environmental pollution of the atmosphere, water or soil. This results from industrial, agricultural and other human activities which has been increasing since the nineteenth century. Human morbidity, mortality and damage to other animals and plants in the environment may result. The *atmosphere* may be polluted by gases such as sulphur and nitrogen oxides and ozone, carbon monoxide, hydrocarbons and *particulates* contributing to smog (reducing and photochemical). Some of these pollutants contribute to **acid rain** and die back of trees. The acidification of lakes and rivers damages aquatic organisms such as salmon and the acid rain damages leaves and leaches essential minerals from the soil. Heavy metals such as **lead** from car exhausts and industrial activity may pollute air, soil and water. Lead causes damage to kidneys, red cells, bones and the nervous system. **Water** may be polluted with industrial, domestic or agricultural waste which can lead to overgrowth of algae and then *eutrophication* or direct toxic effects. Ground water in some countries may be polluted with **arsenic** leading to cancer and skin diseases. A variety of pollutants (e.g. alkylphenols, DDT, PCBs) and fungal products are known to be **endocrine disruptors** which can cause dysfunction of the reproductive system in animals (e.g. alligators, dog whelks, fish) as a result of oestrogenic, anti-oestrogenic or anti-androgenic activity. Humans may be affected (e.g. low sperm counts) but the link is not proven.

Environmental pollutants, particularly if lipophilic (e.g. DDT, dieldrin), may accumulate in organisms and those animals at the top of the **food chain** (e.g. predators) may be exposed to much higher concentrations than exist in the environment (bioaccumulation). **Mercury**, an important pollutant, exists in three forms (organic, elemental or inorganic), all toxic. It contaminated factory effluent which was allowed to pollute the waters of a bay in Japan (Minamata), bioaccumulated in fish and caused death and disease (e.g. birth defects) in many people exposed. Pollutant chemicals now require testing for their potential impact on the environment (BOD, COD) and organisms in it (e.g. *Daphnia*, earthworms).

Questions

Q1. Indicate which of the following is true: Lead:

   a   is toxic because it inhibits mitochondrial respiration
   b   is present in cigarette smoke
   c   damages red blood cells
   d   is not toxic to the nervous system
   e   can be absorbed through the lungs.

Q2. Which of the following statements is not true?

   a   metallic mercury is non-toxic
   b   organic mercury is toxic to the kidney
   c   inorganic mercury is toxic to the brain
   d   inorganic mercury binds to SH groups
   e   methylmercury has a half-life of 70 days.

Q3. Indicate which of the following statements is true:

   a   the great smog in London was in 1852
   b   photochemical smog contains only nitrogen oxides
   c   ozone is a non-toxic gas that promotes good health
   d   PM10 means a concentration of oxidants of $10\ \mu g\,m^{-3}$
   e   acid rain is formed from chlorinated hydrocarbons interacting with the ozone layer
   f   reducing smog has a high level of sulphur dioxide and particulates.

Q4. Indicate which of the following statements is true:
The effect of DDT on the bird population was due to:

a the toxicity of DDT to chicks
b loss of tree cover due to its herbicidal action
c damage to eggs by DDE
d migration
e loss of insects.

SHORT ANSWER QUESTION

Q5. Define the terms *bioaccumulation* and *biomagnification* and state their importance in toxicology. Using one or more suitable examples, describe the properties that chemicals must possess for bioaccumulation.

Bibliography

BARLTROP, D. (1985) Lead and brain damage, *Human Toxicology*, **4**, 121.

BOWN, W. (1994) Dying from too much dust, *New Scientist*, **141** (1916), 12–13.

Casarett and Doull's Toxicology, The Basic Science of Poisons, C. D. Klaassen (Ed.), 5th edition, 1996, New York: McGraw-Hill. Various chapters.

FRANCIS, B. M. (1994) *Toxic Substances in the Environment. An Overview of Environmental Toxicology*. New York: John Wiley.

General and Applied Toxicology, Ballantyne, B., Marrs, T. and Syversen, T.L. (Eds), 2nd edition, 1999, Basingstoke: Macmillan. Various chapters.

MORIARTY, F. (1999) *Ecotoxicology: The Study of Pollutants in Ecosystems*, 3rd edition, London: Academic Press.

OWENS, R. V. and OWENS, R. (1983) *Acidification of the Environment Including Acid Rain*, Powys: Pyramid.

PEAKALL, D. B. (1994) Biomarkers: the way forward in environmental assessment, *Toxicology and Ecotoxicology News*, **1**, 55–60.

PEARCE, F. (1987) Acid rain, *New Scientist*, 5 November, 1–4.

RAND, G. M. (Ed.) (1995) *Fundamentals of Aquatic Toxicology*, 2nd edition, London: Taylor & Francis.

SHAW, I. C. and CHADWICK, J. (1998) *Principles of Environmental Toxicology*, London: Taylor & Francis.

WALKER, C. H., HOPKIN, S. P., SIBLY, R. M. and PEAKALL, D. B. (2001) *Principles of Ecotoxicology*, 2nd edition, London: Taylor & Francis.

ZAKREWSKI, S. F. (1991) *Principles of Environmental Toxicology*, Washington, DC: American Chemical Society.

CHAPTER 10

Natural products

Chapter outline

This chapter considers various specific examples of naturally occuring toxins.

- Plant toxins
    - pyrrolizidine alkaloids
    - pennyroyal oil
    - ricin
    - bracken
    - fluoroacetate
- Animal toxins
    - snake venoms
    - tetrodotoxin
- Fungal toxins
    - Death Cap mushroom
    - aflatoxins
- Microbial toxins
    - botulism and botulinum toxin

Although many of the toxic chemicals in the environment that worry the general public are man-made, there are also many hundreds of natural poisons of animal, plant, fungal and microbial origin. Indeed, the *most toxic* substances known to man are natural poisons such as **botulinum toxin** (Table 1.1) and it is certainly not reasonable to imply, as do some of the advertisements for health foods and herbal medicines, that natural substances are intrinsically harmless and safe. For example, allergies to natural constituents of food are known to occur just as they do to synthetic additives. Some of these natural, toxic substances have been known about for centuries and have been used for murder or suicide, or even sometimes misguided medical treatment (see Chapter 1).

Natural substances also still occasionally feature in accidental poisoning cases although this is relatively rare compared with poisoning by drug overdose. Natural toxins are of diverse structure and mode of action, and there are far too many categories to consider each individually in this book. Consequently we will simply examine a few interesting and important examples of toxic substances derived from plants, animals, fungi and micro-organisms.

Plant toxins

There are many well known plant toxins ranging from the irritant **formic acid** found in nettles (and ants) to more poisonous compounds such as **atropine** in deadly nightshade berries (*Atropa belladonna*), **cytisine** in laburnum and **coniine** in hemlock. Let us consider a few less well-known plant toxins which have been studied recently.

PYRROLIZIDINE ALKALOIDS

Pyrrolizidine alkaloids are a large family of structurally related compounds found in over 6000 plants in the Leguminosae, Compositae and Boraginacae families. Many of these occur as weeds throughout the world. About half of the pyrrolizidine alkaloids have been identified as toxic and these plant constituents are probably the most common cause of poisoning in the world for humans and animals, both livestock and domestic. This may occur as a result of contamination of cereal crops or as a result of use of plants in herbal remedies.

Case study *In Austria an 18-month-old boy presented with veno-occlusive disease. He had been given herbal tea since he was 3 months old. The herbal tea had been intended to have been made with Coltsfoot but was in fact made with Alpendost. The boy had congestion of the sinusoids of the liver and necrosis and bleeding from the small veins.*

A study in South Africa in two hospitals identified 20 children suffering from veno-occlusive disease which was thought to be due to the use of traditional remedies. Most of the children had fluid in the abdominal cavity and an enlarged liver. There was high morbidity and mortality and in those that survived the disease progressed to liver cirrhosis. In four cases pyrrolizidine alkaloids were detected in the urine.

Poisoning has occured in various parts of the world, especially where agricultural conditions are poor and the indigenous population may be forced to use the contaminated crops. For example, in South Africa during the 1930s poor whites suffered the toxic effects of these alkaloids because their staple diet was wheat which became contaminated, whereas their Bantu neighbours, who ate maize which was not contaminated, were not affected. More recently, poisonings have occurred in Tashkent, Central India and Northern Afghanistan. In one incident where 1600 poisoning cases were reported, the threshed wheat was found to be contaminated with ***Heliotropium popovii*** seeds giving an alkaloid concentration of at *least 0.5 per cent*. In the West Indies especially, these plants may also be used in traditional medicine to make herbal teas.

The toxicity depends on the particular alkaloid. One of the most studied pyrrolizidine alkaloids is **monocrotaline**. This is found in *Heliotropium*, *Senecio* and *Crotolaria* species and it causes liver injury in humans, such as after acute exposure to herbal teas for example. The liver injury is of an unusual kind causing damage to the sinusoids in the liver, known as **veno-occlusive disease**.

Monocrotaline will consistently produce veno-occlusive disease in rats and also damage the lungs. The effect of chronic exposure to low doses is **liver cirrhosis** which can be seen in some members of the West Indian population, estimated to account for one third of the cirrhosis seen at autopsy in Jamaica. The constituent

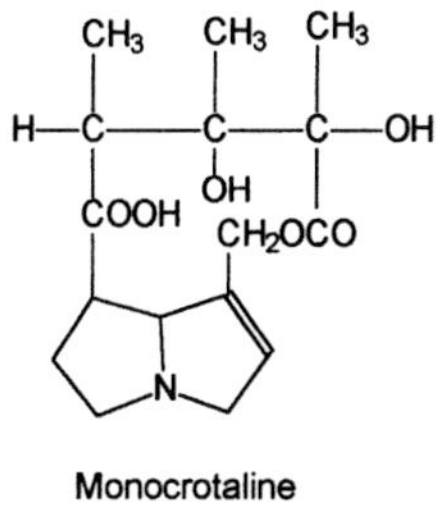

FIGURE 10.1 *The structure of the pyrrolizidine alkaloid monocrotaline.*

alkaloids, such as **monocrotaline** (Figure 10.1), undergo metabolic activation to a reactive metabolite which damages the cells lining the liver sinusoids as well as the hepatocytes, leading to haemorrhagic necrosis and finally to the **veno-occlusive disease**. This blockage of the blood vessels in the liver eventually gives rise to alteration of the vasculature such that the liver blood supply is diverted and new blood vessels grow.

Animals may also be exposed and suffer the toxic effects. Where there is abundant vegetation for grazing, animals will ignore plants such as **ragwort (*Senecio jacoboea*)** which contain the alkaloids but in some countries, such as Australia, widespread losses of horses, cattle and sheep have occurred from *Heliotropium* poisoning. This may also be another route of human exposure as the alkaloids can be detected in the milk of cows grazing on such plants.

PENNYROYAL OIL

The Pennyroyal plant and the oil prepared from it have been used to induce abortions in the USA where it is possible to buy the oil 'over the counter'. The plant may be used to make a tea or the oil may be taken directly. Both may cause toxic effects, especially liver damage as well as inducing abortion. The oil contains a number of terpenoid compounds and metabolic activation is believed to be required for the toxicity.

RICIN

Ricin is a highly toxic plant product found in the seeds of the castor oil plant. It achieved some notoriety when it was claimed that it had been used by the Bulgarian secret police to kill the Bulgarian journalist **Georgi Markov** in London in 1978. Although no trace of any poison was found in the victim's body clearly an extremely potent poison had been used and the symptoms were consistent with those of ricin poisoning. A tiny metal pellet was recovered from a wound on the victim's leg, seemingly inflicted accidentally by an umbrella. The pellet almost certainly was a reservoir for a toxic substance, but it could only contain a few nanograms of the substance.

Ricin is a small **protein** consisting of **two polypeptides**, a short A chain and a longer B chain. The A and B chains are linked via a disulphide bridge. The B chain attaches the ricin molecule to the outside of the mammalian cell by binding to the galactose part of a glycoprotein. The cell membrane invaginates and the ricin is taken into the cell inside a vacuole. The ricin molecule is released from the glycoprotein and the A and B chains then break at the disulphide bridge. The B chain makes a channel through the vacuole cell wall, allowing the A chain to enter the cytoplasm and reach the ribosomes where it blocks protein synthesis and kills the cell. One molecule of ricin is sufficient to kill one cell.

BRACKEN

The bracken fern contains a substance, **ptaquiloside**, which degrades into a compound which is carcinogenic. In Japan, the shoots of the bracken fern are eaten and this may explain the high incidence of throat cancer among the Japanese. Animals which eat the fern as fodder suffer from bladder and intestinal cancer. The breakdown product of ptaquiloside reacts with DNA, specifically the base adenine, and this is lost with the result that the DNA chain breaks.

FLUOROACETATE

For a description of the toxicity of this naturally occurring plant toxin see Chapter 8.

There are many more well-known substances derived from plants such as the drugs **heroin, morphine, cannabis, nicotine** and **digitalis**.

Animal toxins

As with plant toxins, animal toxins comprise a diverse range of structures and modes of action (Figure 10.2). A simple and well-known example is formic acid which is found in ants (the name is derived from the Latin word, *formica*, for an ant). Other examples are **tetrodotoxin** found in the **Puffer Fish** and **saxitoxin** found in shellfish and fish which have consumed certan dinoflagellates. Animal toxins are often mixtures of **complex proteins**. Most of us suffer

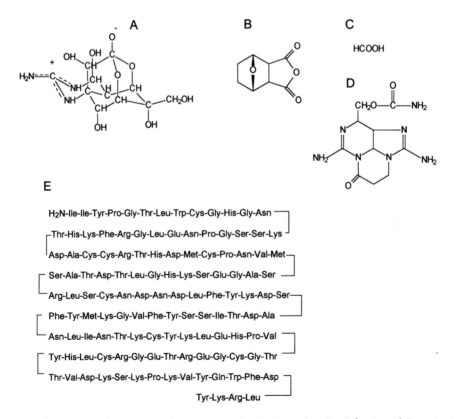

FIGURE 10.2 *The structures of various animal toxins. A: tetrodotoxin; B: cantharidin; C: formic acid; D: saxitoxin; E: amino acid sequence from honey bee venom phospholipase A.*

from animal toxins at some time in our lives even if it is only a wasp or bee sting. However, in some countries death and illness due to animal poisons represents an important proportion of poisoning cases and a significant cause of illness and death.

SNAKE VENOMS

Snake bites are one of the most common forms of poisoning by natural toxins worldwide. Many snake venoms are similar in their mode of action and constituents, being mixtures of **proteins or polypeptides**. The proteins may be enzymes, especially **hydrolytic enzymes**. Some of the more important are **proteinases, phospholipases, ribonucleases, deoxyribonucleases, phosphomonoesterases** and **phosphodiesterases**, and **ATPases**. The toxicity of some snake venoms is shown in Table 10.1. The venoms may be mixtures and consequently cause a variety of effects. For example, the presence of foreign proteins may cause an **anaphylactic reaction**, although this is rare, and such allergic reactions may cause death in minutes. The enzyme components can *digest* various tissue constituents either at the site of action, causing local necrosis, or elsewhere causing systemic effects. For example, the bite of the diamondback rattle-snake, the most poisonous snake in the USA, produces a very painful swelling within minutes. Nausea, vomiting and diarrhoea may occur and cardiac effects, such as a *fall* in systemic arterial blood pressure and a weak, rapid pulse, may be seen. The central nervous system can be affected, leading to respiratory paralysis. Haemolytic anaemia and haemoglobinuria sometimes occur, and there may be thrombosis and haemorrhage. Vascular permeability and nerve conduction can change, and cerebral anoxia, pulmonary oedema and heart failure also develop. The **phospholipases** found in snake venom sometimes cause *intravascular haemolysis* by direct action on the red cell membrane.

Most snake venoms contain a **phosphodiesterase** which *attacks* polynucleotides.

TETRODOTOXIN

This toxin is found in the **Puffer Fish** and also in the **Californian newt** and bacteria and has been studied extensively. The fish is eaten as a delicacy in Japan and provided it is properly prepared is edible and safe. However, fatalities have occurred which resulted from incorrect preparation of the fish and about *60 per cent of poisoning cases are fatal*. The tetrodotoxin and another

TABLE 10.1 *Comparative toxicity of snake venoms*

Snake venom	Yield (g)	LD$_{50}$ i.v. mg kg^{-1}
Copperhead	40–72	10.92
African puff adder	130–200	3.68
Mojave rattler	50–90	0.21
Russell's viper	130–250	0.08
Sea snake	7–20	0.01

Source: F. W. Oehme, J. F. Brown and M. E. Fowler (1980), Toxins of animal origin, in *Casarett and Doull's Toxicology*, J. Doull, C. D. Klaassen and M. O. Amdur (Eds), 2nd edition, New York: Macmillan.

toxin **ichthyocrinotoxin** are found in the roe, liver and skin of the fish. Tetrodotoxin is a very potent nerve poison, lethal at doses of around 10 μg kg^{-1} body weight. Initial effects are a tingling in the mouth followed within 10–45 minutes by muscular incoordination, salivation, skin numbness, vomiting, diarrhoea and convulsions. Death results from skeletal muscle paralysis. Sensory as well as motor nerves are affected and it is believed that tetrodotoxin *selectively blocks* the **sodium channels** along the axon, preventing the inward action potential current.

Fungal toxins

Many fungi produce toxins of a variety of chemical types and these can cause acute or chronic poisoning. Poisonous mushrooms may be confused with the edible varieties and hence accidental acute poisoning may occur. Poisoning may also occur through the intentional eating of fungi believed to contain psychoactive substances. Several fungal toxins have been fully identified and characterized. The toxic effects vary from relatively mild gastrointestinal disturbances to severe organ damage. Some, such as the psychoactive constituents **mescaline** and **psilocin**, affect the central nervous system. Certain fungal products, such as the **aflatoxins** which are discussed in Chapter 7, are potent **carcinogens**.

DEATH CAP MUSHROOM

The Death Cap mushroom, ***Amanita phalloides*** is probably the most poisonous mushroom in Britain. It is occasionally eaten by mistake, but poisoning with this mushroom is rare in the UK. The mushroom contains a number of toxins: the phallotoxins, including **phal-** **loidin**, **phalloin** and **phallolysin**, and the **amatoxins** (α, β and γ amanitin). The phallotoxins cause violent **gastroenteritis** which occurs rapidly (4–8 hours) after the mushroom is eaten.

The amatoxins have a delayed toxic effect, with the liver and kidney as target organs; **liver necrosis** and **destruction of renal tubular cells** may result. Both the phallotoxins and the amanitins are strongly bound to plasma proteins yet are toxic in this form. Consequently, treatment involves *displacement* from the proteins by a drug such as a **sulphonamide** or **benzylpenicillin** which will reduce toxicity. This is probably due to increased excretion of the unbound form as protein binding of foreign compounds slows excretion (see Chapter 2).

After the mushroom is eaten sometimes there may not be any symptoms for up to a day then vomiting and diarrhoea occur possibly followed by jaundice, hypoglycaemia, acidosis and other effects on blood chemistry. In severe cases hepatic failure can result.

AFLATOXINS

These fungal toxins have already been discussed under food contaminants (Chapter 8). **Aflatoxin B$_1$** causes **liver damage** after high doses but in humans chronic exposure to lower doses via the diet is a more likely occurrence which can cause **liver tumours**. The toxin is most likely to occur in food infected with the mould ***Aspergillus flavus*** or prepared from infected food or ingredients.

Microbial toxins

There are many toxins produced by bacteria. As with other natural toxins, they are of a variety of chemical types and consequently they cause a variety of different toxic effects, ranging from gastrointestinal effects to severe and fatal effects on the nervous system. We will consider just one well known toxic syndrome, botulism.

BOTULISM AND BOTULINUM TOXIN

Botulinum toxin is a toxicant derived from a spore forming anaerobic bacterium, *Clostridium botulinum*. The bacterium produces a mixture of six **neurotoxic proteins** and poisoning with these toxins causes a syndrome, botulism, which has a high mortality rate. The toxin is one of the most toxic substances known to man with an LD_{50} of around 0.01 μg kg^{-1} and so less than a microgram would be lethal for a human. The spores are quite resistant but the toxin is destroyed by heat (80°C). The symptoms of poisoning normally appear 18–36 hours after ingestion although the appearance may be as short as 4 hours or as long as 4 days.

The mechanism underlying the effect of botulinum toxin is irreversible blockade of the motor nerve terminal at the **myoneural junction**, preventing the release of acetylcholine. The result is that the muscle behaves as if it is denervated and the victim suffers paralysis. This leads to weakness of limbs and difficulty in breathing which may be fatal if severe. There is fortunately an anti-toxin available.

Although cases of botulism are thankfully rare, they still occur from time to time, sometimes affecting several victims at the same time as a result of contaminated food. This is typically home-canned food such as seafood, vegetables, sausages and other meat products, which have not been adequately preserved or refrigerated.

Case study *In October and November 1987 eight cases of botulism occurred, two in New York and six in Israel. All of the victims had* *eaten Kapchunka, air-dried, salted whitefish, which had been prepared in New York and some transported by individuals to Israel. All the patients developed the symptoms of botulism within 36 hours and one died. Some were treated with anti-toxin and two received breathing assistance.*

Summary and learning objectives

There are thousands of chemicals found naturally in the environment in plants, fungi, bacteria and animals and a significant number are toxic. For example, ***pyrrolizidine alkaloids*** such as monocrotaline, found in plants such as *Senecio* and *Heliotropium*, cause poisoning (liver damage) in animals and humans as a result of contamination of crops or use as herbal remedies. ***Pennyroyal oil***, from the Pennyroyal plant and used to induce abortions in the USA, causes liver damage. ***Ricin*** from the castor oil plant, is a protein and the most toxic substance known. ***Ptaquiloside*** found in the ***bracken*** fern is a carcinogen in both humans and animals. ***Animal toxins*** such as ***snake venoms*** generally consist of a variety of hydrolytic enzyme toxins (e.g. proteinases, phosphoesterases) which may cause anaphylactic shock as well as tissue necrosis. ***Tetrodotoxin***, found in Puffer Fish and bacteria, is a potent nerve poison. Phalloidin from the ***Death Cap mushroom***, contains several toxins that damage liver and kidneys. Another fungal toxin is ***aflatoxin*** from *Aspergillus flavus*. ***Botulinum toxin*** from the bacterium *Clostridium botulinum*, consists of neurotoxic proteins which are extremely potent, causing irreversible blockade of the myoneural junction. Poisoning may often result in paralysis and fatal respiratory failure.

Questions

Q1. Indicate which of the following are true:

a pyrrolizidine alkaloids are found in mushrooms

b *Amanita phalloides* is a poisonous snake

c Botulinum toxin is produced by bacteria

d ricin is the toxin in puffer fish

e fluoroacetate is a plant toxin.

Q2. Which of the following statements about tetrodoxin are true:

a it is a toxin found in blue green algae

b it causes paralysis of muscles in humans

c it affects calcium channels

d it blocks nervous transmission.

SHORT ANSWER QUESTION

Q3. What is the basic mechanism underlying the toxicity of botulinum toxin?

Bibliography

Casarett and Doull's Toxicology, The Basic Science of Poisons, C. D. Klaassen (Ed.), 5th edition, 1996, New York: McGraw-Hill. Various chapters.

EMSLEY, J. (1994) How bracken's deadly chemical breaks the back of DNA, *New Scientist*, **142** (1921), 16.

General and Applied Toxicology, Ballantyne, B., Marrs, T. and Syversen, T. L. M. (Eds), 2nd edition, 1999, Basingstoke: Macmillan. Various chapters.

HABERMEYL, G. G. (1981) *Venomous Animals and Their Toxins,* Berlin: Springer Verlag.

HARRIS, J. B. (Ed.) (1986) *Natural Toxins, Animal, Plant and Microbial,* Oxford: Oxford University Press.

HMSO (1987) Mycotoxins, Food Surveillance Paper no. 18, London: HMSO.

MANN, J. (1994) *Murder, Magic and Medicine*, Oxford University Press. A readable book with much interesting historical information.

MATOSSIAN, M. K. (1989) *Poisons of the Past; Molds, Epidemics and History.* Yale University Press. An interesting and readable historical book.

MEBS, D. (2001) Toxicity in animals: trends in evolution? *Toxicon*, **39**, 87.

MOFFAT, A. C. (1980) Forensic pharmacognosy – poisoning with plants, *Journal of Forensic Science Society*, **20**, 103.

RECHCIGL, M. (Ed.) (1983) *Handbook of Naturally Occurring Food Toxicants,* Boca Raton: CRC Press.

TWIGG, L. E. and KING, D. R. (1991) The impact of fluoroacetate-bearing vegetation on native Australian fauna: a review, *Oikos*, **61**, 412–430.

CHAPTER — **11**

Household products

Chapter outline

In this chapter some examples of poisoning with household products and miscellaneous chemicals and treatment of poisoning will be considered:

- Introduction
- Carbon monoxide
- Antifreeze: ethylene glycol
- Cyanide
- Alcohol
- Glue sniffing and solvent abuse
- Treatment of poisoning and antidotes

Introduction

This group of potential poisons comprises many substances, some of which fit into one or more of the other categories already dis-

cussed. For example, the herbicide **paraquat** (see Chapter 8) is widely used by domestic gardeners as well as by horticulturalists, and consequently it is often found in the home. Drugs too are often found around the household, however, these have been discussed already and will not be further mentioned.

Household products feature in poisoning cases usually after accidental ingestion by children and occasionally in suicide cases. The majority of enquiries relating to childhood poisoning, especially in children under 5-years-old, are in connection with non-medicinal, mainly household products or toxic substances to which people may be exposed in the home. However, the number of deaths due to substances used in the home is small, six in the UK in 1978 and 21 in the USA in 1976. Many deaths in children under 10-years of age and adults are due to **carbon monoxide** and consequently this will be discussed in detail.

Some of the potentially toxic substances found in the home are corrosive and some are generally only ingested intentionally. **Bleach** is perhaps the substance most commonly involved in poisoning cases. Other substances include strong **detergents** such as dishwasher powder, **drain cleaners** which are generally **caustic** (i.e. corrosive), and **kettle descalers** which are *corrosive* (Figure 11.1). When bleach is ingested orally it causes burning to the throat, mouth and oesophagus. The tissue damage results in *oedema* in the pharynx and larynx. In the stomach the presence of endogenous hydrochloric acid generates hypochlorous acid which is an *irritant*, and chlorine gas which may be inhaled causing toxic effects in, and damage to, the lungs. However, serious injury from ingestion of bleach rarely occurs as it requires relatively large quantities and this is usually intentional rather than accidental.

Hydrocarbon solvents such as turpentine substitute and white spirit are often used for cleaning paint brushes. They may be dangerous by aspiration which can lead to a chemical **pneumonitis**. Having a low viscosity and being volatile, the solvent spreads through the lungs easily and therefore can affect a large area.

Carbon monoxide

This highly toxic gas is still a major cause of poisoning deaths in the UK despite the fact that a major source, coal gas, has been replaced by natural gas. Several hundred deaths occur annually and carbon monoxide poisoning is still a major cause of death from poisoning in children. The gas is found in **car exhausts** and results from the inefficient burning of hydrocarbon fuels in engines as well as in **stoves** and **boilers** especially where there is poor ventilation. There have, in fact, been a number of poisonings recently, some with fatal outcomes which have been highlighted in the press and on television in the UK. In one recent case, a birds nest had blocked the chimney of a holiday cottage and so when the

AYLESBURY PLUS, WEDNESDAY, SEPTEMBER 16 1987

Agonising death of haunted woman

A HAUNTED Wendover woman died an agonising death after drinking kettle descaler.

In the last year Mrs Heidi Mason, 44, of Orchard Close, Wendover, had tried to kill herself with pill overdoses, a razor blade and a plastic bag after becoming a victim of serious depression.

She was found, bleeding from the mouth, half-conscious but dying, in the grounds of St John's psychiatric hospital, Stone, where she was a voluntary patient, on June 4.

Her stomach was almost entirely eaten away by the acid and her mouth and throat badly blistered.

But despite her history of suicide attempts, Bucks coroner Rodney Corner refused to record a verdict of suicide at Mrs Mason's inquest in Aylesbury on Friday.

He recorded an open verdict, saying he could not be certain she had intended to kill herself this time.

Dr Julian Candy, psychologist at St John's, told the inquest that Mrs Mason believed that people around her knew certain things about her past.

'Mrs Mason suffered from self-blame, guilt and depression, and discussed suicide with me on several occasions,' said Dr Candy.

'She had an intense feeling of hopelessness. A number of deaths in the family including her mother's and stepfather's caused her great distress.'

Pathologist Dr Andrew Tudway said that Mrs Mason's stomach was almost entirely corroded and her mouth and throat ulcerated by the formic acid in the kettle descaler.

FIGURE 11.1 *A headline reminds us of the potential toxicity of household substances. In this case, kettle descaler containing corrosive formic acid was taken intentionally. Taken from the newspaper,* Aylesbury Plus, *16 September 1987, with permission.*

fire was lit, the lack of ventilation caused the fire to produce carbon monoxide. All the members of the family subsequently died in the house from carbon monoxide poisoning (see Emsley, Bibliography).

Carbon monoxide is a very simple poison and its mode of action has been understood for many years. Poisoning with it is also relatively simple to treat. In 1895 **Haldane** conducted experiments with carbon monoxide using himself as a subject. He carefully documented the effects as the concentration of carbon monoxide in his blood stream rose towards lethal levels. Through his studies and the earlier work of **Claude Bernard** in 1865 we now know much about the mechanism of action of carbon monoxide as a poison.

Carbon monoxide reacts with the **haemoglobin** in red blood cells. It does this by binding to the iron atom of the haem molecule in the same way as oxygen (Figure 11.2). Carbon monoxide binds *more avidly* than oxygen, however, and the resulting carboxyhaemoglobin cannot carry out its normal function of transporting oxygen. Therefore, there is competition for binding to haemoglobin between oxygen and carbon monoxide and the concentration of the latter is a crucial factor. As carbon monoxide binds much more avidly to the iron atom the concentration of the toxic gas necessary to saturate the

haemoglobin is much less than that of oxygen in air. This was determined by Haldane and is shown by his equation:

$$\frac{[COHb]}{[HbO_2]} = \frac{M[P_{CO}]}{[P_{O2}]}$$

where **M is 220**, at pH 7.4 in man. [COHb] and [HbO$_2$] are the concentration of carboxyhaemoglobin and haemoglobin respectively. [Pco] and [P$_{O2}$] are the partial pressures of carbon monoxide and oxygen respectively.

Consequently, for 50 per cent saturation of haemoglobin with carbon monoxide, where 50 per cent of the haemoglobin in the blood is carboxyhaemoglobin, the concentration of carbon monoxide need only be *1/220* of that of oxygen in the air or about *0.1 per cent*. A level of 50 per cent carboxyhaemoglobin would certainly be lethal for a human after a relatively short time. As carbon monoxide is also *odourless* and *tasteless*, it is an extremely dangerous poison. The result of carbon monoxide poisoning is that the tissues are starved of oxygen and suffer **ischaemic damage**. Energy production is reduced, only anaerobic respiration being possible and, hence, there is an accumulation of lactic acid causing **acidosis**.

The symptoms of carbon monoxide poisoning depend on the concentration to which the victim is exposed. There is often **headache, mental confusion, agitation, nausea and vomiting**. The skin becomes characteristically pink due to the carboxyhaemoglobin in the blood. The victim hyperventilates and will eventually lose consciousness and suffer **respiratory failure**. There may be **brain** and **cardiac damage** resulting from the hypoxia, and also **cardiac arrythmias** and other malfunctions of the heart can occur.

Treatment is relatively simple, especially for mild cases and involves removing the victim from the source of carbon monoxide, or causing fresh uncontaminated air to be introduced into

FIGURE 11.2 *The haem moiety of the haemoglobin molecule showing the binding of the oxygen molecule to the iron atom. As shown in the diagram, carbon monoxide (CO) binds at the same site as the oxygen molecule, but it is bound much more tightly. (His is the side chain of the amino acid Histidine.)*

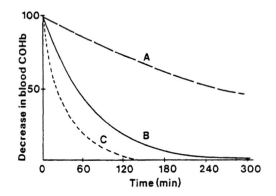

FIGURE 11.3 *The dissociation of carboxyhaemoglobin in the bloodstream of a patient poisoned with carbon monoxide. The graphs show the effects of breathing air (A), oxygen (B) or oxygen at increased pressure (2.5 atmospheres) (C) on the rate of dissociation.* Data from Meredith, T. J. and Vale, J. A. (1981), Antidotes, pp. 33–45, Figure 5.9, in Poisoning – Diagnosis and Treatment, J. A. Vale and T. J. Meredith (Eds), London: Update Books.

the immediate environment. As the concentration of carbon monoxide in the ambient air and hence the inspired air falls, the carboxyhaemoglobin dissociates and the carbon monoxide is expired. This rate of loss of carbon monoxide from the blood (half-life around 250 minutes) can be *increased* by making the patient breathe oxygen rather than air (half-life reduced to 50 minutes). For severe poisoning cases the use of oxygen at *elevated pressures* (2.5 atmospheres) will reduce the half-life of elimination to around 22 minutes (Figure 11.3). The reductions in half-life with oxygen at elevated concentrations and pressures can be predicted from the Haldane equation.

Antifreeze: ethylene glycol

Antifreeze liquid contains one or sometimes two toxic compounds which may feature in poi-soning, either accidental or suicidal. The major constituent of antifreeze is ethylene glycol but this may sometimes be combined with **methanol**.

Ethylene glycol is a dihydric alcohol and a sweet tasting liquid, which has effects on the state of mind similar to those of ethanol. It may sometimes be consumed instead of normal alcohol by alcoholics. It is very toxic, however, and fatal poisoning may occur after as little as a cupful of antifreeze.

It is not intrinsically toxic but requires *metabolism*. There are various intermediate metabolic products terminating in **oxalic acid** (Figure 3.2). The intermediate acidic metabolites cause **acidosis** directly and also by increasing the level of NADH which is then utilized in the production of lactic acid. As well as being acidic, oxalic acid damages the brain by crystallizing there. **Calcium oxalate crystals** may also form in the kidney tubules and cause damage.

The first step in the metabolism of ethylene glycol involves the enzyme **alcohol dehydrogenase** and this provides the key to the treatment of poisoning. The preferred substrate for this enzyme is ethanol and so when ethanol is present *in vivo* it is *preferentially* metabolized. The metabolism of ethylene glycol is therefore *blocked*. The treatment for ethylene glycol poisoning is, therefore, administration of **ethanol** (whisky or some similar spirit in an emergency) by mouth or pure ethanol can be infused intravenously until all of the ethylene glycol has been excreted from the body. **Haemoperfusion** or **haemodialysis** may also be used to remove ethylene glycol from the body.

The Austrian wine scandal of 1986 involved ethylene glycol being used to sweeten the wine. The amounts used however would not have been acutely toxic although the chronic toxic effects of ethylene glycol, deposition of calcium oxalate kidney stones, might have been a cause for concern. The fact that wine also contains ethanol raises the interesting possibility that the toxicity would be reduced by the continued presence of the antidote!

Methanol, which may sometimes be present in antifreeze, is also found in **methylated spirits** (industrial spirit). It is also very toxic due to its metabolism to **formaldehyde** and **formic acid**:

$$CH_3OH \rightarrow HCHO \rightarrow HCOOH$$

The former may cause **blindness** if the dose of methanol is not rapidly fatal. Again, as methanol is metabolized by alcohol dehydrogenase, treatment of poisoning involves administration of **ethanol** and correction of metabolic acidosis, in the same way as for ethylene glycol poisoning. It may be that the presence of large amounts of ethanol in methylated spirits confers some protection on those unfortunates who drink it either accidentally or intentionally as a substitute for alcoholic drinks.

Cyanide

Cyanides of various kinds are found both naturally in the environment and as a result of human activity. Cyanide is often associated with homicidal or suicidal poisoning and there are some well known cases, but there are many ways in which humans can be exposed. For example, fatalities in fires may result from cyanide poisoning because certain substances, such as plastics, generate **HCN** gas when burning. Cyanides are extensively used in the metal industry and in mining for the extraction of gold, for example. Therefore there is potential for occupational poisoning and contamination of the environment with cyanides. Indeed, there are several documented cases of pollution of rivers from mining operations. In February 2000 a serious case of river pollution occurred in Romania where cyanide from a mining

operation leaked into the river Tiza destroying most of the fish and then as it moved down the river it also destroyed many fish in the rivers and tributaries in Hungary. Inorganic cyanides are often found in laboratories and were once used around the home for the removal of pests such as wasps nests.

Naturally occurring cyanides, such as **amygdalin**, which is a **cyanogenic glycoside**, are found in the kernels and pips of fruits such as apricots, peaches and apples. The most significant natural source of cyanide, however, is **Cassava** which is an important food crop eaten in Africa. The Cassava plant has to be prepared with care in order to avoid poisoning with cyanide. This is usually done by washing and soaking the plant in water. This allows the enzymes in the plant to degrade the cyanogenic glycoside, **Linamarin**, and then the water soluble cyanide ion is washed out. If this is not done and the plant is eaten without this careful preparation, then the cyanogenic glycosides can be degraded by the enzymes in the human gut and the cyanide released in sufficient quantities to poison the unfortunate person who eats the plant.

Hydrogen cyanide is rapidly fatal when inhaled as a vapour but a dose of about 300 mg sodium or potassium cyanide when taken by mouth might take some time to kill the victim depending on factors such as the presence of food in the gut.

The mechanism by which cyanide is toxic involves inhibition of the respiratory chain in the mitochondria. The cyanide binds to **cytochrome aa$_3$** and blocks the movement of electrons down the respiratory chain (Figure 11.4). This means that cellular metabolism is compromised and ATP production is drastically reduced, although not stopped completely. Organs such as the brain and heart are affected particularly as they require ATP and have limited capacity to cope with a deficit. The heart has only enough ATP to last three

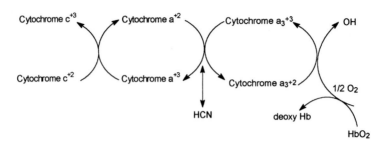

FIGURE 11.4 *The site of action of cyanide in the mitochondrial electron transport chain. Hb: haemoglobin; HbO₂:*
oxyhaemoglobin.

minutes and so cyanide may cause death as a result of heart or respiratory failure. There are several antidotes to cyanide poisoning. One method of treatment is to boost detoxication by giving the patient **thiosulphate** which is involved in an endogenous reaction catalysed by the enzyme **rhodanese**. This converts cyanide into thiocyanate which is less toxic and is excreted into the urine. Increasing the availability of thiosulphate increases the capacity of this reaction to detoxify cyanide. Other methods of treatment involve the use of substances to remove the cyanide such as chelating agents like **dicobalt edetate** (see antidotes, this chapter).

Chronic, non-fatal exposure to cyanide such as that which occurs as a result of eating Cassava may cause other pathological effects such as paralysis due to damage to the spinal cord. This is a significant toxic effect in some parts of Africa where Cassava is a staple diet. An additional factor in the poisoning is the poor diet in parts of Africa where Cassava is eaten which means that local people may be deficient in sulphur amino acids and hence have low levels of thiosulphate. Consequently, they are less able to detoxify the cyanide. A secondary effect is **goitre** (enlarged thyroid) due to the thiocyanate detoxication product of cyanide causing interference in the uptake of iodine essential for the function of the thyroid.

Alcohol

Ethanol is perhaps our most ubiquitous drug and features in far more cases of poisoning or adverse effects than more notorious drugs such as heroin or cocaine. Many members of the general public probably do not consider alcohol to be a drug but it has both *pharmacological* and *toxic* effects. The effects of ethanol vary with the dose and there is some evidence that it may even have beneficial effects at low doses (see Saul, Bibliography). Ethanol is rapidly absorbed from the gut and distributes into body water. About 90 per cent is metabolized to **acetaldehyde, acetic acid** and then carbon dioxide and water at a rate of 10–20 ml h^{-1}. After acute doses the major effect of ethanol is **depression of the central nervous system**. The pharmacological effects may be desirable if the dose is low but after higher doses the effects become exaggerated, progressing through increasing visual impairment, muscular incoordination and slowed reaction times and after large, toxic doses unconsciousness and death. A lethal dose in an adult is between 300 and 500 ml (equivalent to about a litre of whisky) if taken in less than an hour. Large doses may cause a reversible change in the liver known as **fatty liver** where triglycerides accumulate in the hepatic cells. The effects of ethanol can be related to the plasma level and range from mild intoxication at levels of between 500 and 1500 mg l^{-1} to coma and death at levels of more than 5000 mg l^{-1}. At this level respiratory depression, hypotension, hypothermia and hypoglycaemia will occur. The hypoglycaemia is largely due to the inhibition of gluconeogenesis by ethanol.

After chronic exposure to ethanol the liver is the main target organ although the brain may also suffer. **Cirrhosis** of the liver occurs after chronic abuse of alcohol and in this toxic effect the architecture of the liver is altered by the replacement of normal tissue by collagen so that it *functions less efficiently*. The biochemical basis of the hepatic effects of ethanol are complex and involve alterations in the level of cofactors such as NADH and disturbances in intermediary metabolism. Thus, a *shift* in the **redox potential** with an increased NADH/ NAD ratio leads to impaired mitochondrial oxidation of fatty acids such that more triglyceride is synthesized. Ethanol, however, causes various other metabolic effects which contribute to the toxicity.

Ethanol is now classified as a **carcinogen** from epidemiological evidence in man which associates cancer of the liver and parts of the gastrointestinal tract to its use.

Glue sniffing and solvent abuse

Glue sniffing and solvent abuse became common among teenagers during the 1970s and 1980s. Many different types of solvent were used with correspondingly different effects. **Toluene** is a solvent commonly found in glues and mainly causes **narcosis**. Some of the **halogenated solvents** such as those used as aerosol propellants are more hazardous, as they may cause *sensitization of the myocardium* to catecholamines leading to **ventricular**

arrhythmias. This effect can lead to sudden death from **heart attack**, especially under certain conditions such as fright, and over 120 deaths occurred in the UK in 1991. Solvents are found in many different household products including glues, paints, paint strippers, aerosols, varnishes, cleaning fluids and fire extinguishers and so the scope for abuse is enormous. The acute toxic effects of solvents are mainly narcosis or anaesthesia and the more serious sensitization of the heart. The chronic effects are in many cases unknown but may include changes in personality and general morbidity. There are, however, known cases of chronic cardiac toxicity due to **trichloroethane** exposure.

Antidotes and the treatment of poisoning

This section is relevant to a number of the examples and substances covered in various chapters and consequently is placed in this penultimate chapter of the book.

Poisoning of humans may result from the accidental or intentional overdosage with drugs or other chemicals. This usually, but not always, follows oral ingestion and is normally an acute poisoning episode. Such poisoning requires treatment and falls within the remit of clinical toxicology. However, repeated or chronic exposure may lead to acute poisoning, and exposure via inhalation or skin absorption can also feature in acute poisoning cases.

For some chemicals there are specific antidotes which can be administered, and which reduce the toxicity of the substance swallowed. There are, however, relatively few of these. In most cases poisoning is treated by means other than the use of antidotes.

GENERAL METHODS

1 One of the most common general methods for the treatment of poisoning is the use of substances to remove the toxicant from the gastrointestinal tract. This can be done in one of two ways:

a Use of **emetics**. These substances cause the poisoned patient to vomit and so eject the poison from the gastrointestinal tract. **Syrup of Ipecachuana** is one such emetic which can be used in children.

b The use of **absorbants**. Absorbants such as **Fullers Earth** or activated charcoal remove the substance from the gastrointestinal tract by absorption and strong binding. This treatment is effective for many different types of poisons.

2 Another commonly used general method of treatment is to increase elimination from the body. This can be done by changing the acidity or alkalinity of the urine or by simply increasing the urine flow. The urine flow is increased by making the patient imbibe large amounts of water or by injecting fluid intravenously. So-called **forced diuresis** is not without hazard, however. Increasing the elimination by changing the acidity or alkalinity of the urine is effective for drugs and chemicals or their metabolites which are charged, i.e. acids or bases. The basis of this is that acids will be more soluble in urine which has an alkaline pH and vice versa, bases will be more soluble in acidic urine. Changing the urine to a more alkaline pH can be achieved by giving the poisoned patient **sodium bicarbonate** either orally or by intravenous injection. This is used effectively with **aspirin** poisoning (see Chapter 5) or **barbiturate poisoning**. Conversely, the urine may be acidified by giving the patient **ammonium chloride**. This may be used for the treatment of **amphetamine** poisoning. As well as increasing elimination into the urine this technique also changes the pH of the plasma which may increase distribution of the drug out of the tissues into the blood. This occurs in the case of both phenobarbital and salicylic acid, which being acidic, become more ionized in the plasma as the pH rises. The ionized forms of these drugs are less able to penetrate the tissues, especially the brain, thereby reducing the toxicity.

3 Drugs and toxicants can also be directly removed from the blood by the techniques of **haemodialysis** and **haemoperfusion**. Both involve the passage of the blood of the poisoned patient through an apparatus which either allows diffusion of the toxicant through a semi-permeable membrane into another fluid (haemodialysis) or removes the toxicant from the blood by adsorption onto charcoal or a resin (haemoperfusion).

ANTIDOTES

Antidotes act in various ways but there are few in relation to the number of toxicants available. Antidotes can act in one of a number of ways.

1 **Chelating agents**. These act by reacting with the compound to form a water soluble complex which can be eliminated. The toxicant is thereby removed from the body. Examples of chelating agents used for the treatment of poisoning are **dicobalt edetate** used for the treatment of cyanide poisoning (see this chapter), penicillamine used for treating lead poisoning (see Chapter 9) and **dimercaprol** used against the poison

gas Lewisite and also for heavy metal poisoning.

2 Antidotes which specifically **increase** the **detoxication** of a reactive metabolite. A good example of this is **N-acetylcysteine**, used for the treatment of paracetamol overdoses (see Chapter 5). N-acetylcysteine increases the detoxication of the reactive metabolite of paracetamol (p-benzoquinoneimine) by increasing the production of glutathione. Therefore the reactive metabolite is diverted away from the toxic interaction with liver protein and the toxicity is reduced. Stimulation of the detoxication of cyanide by increasing its metabolic conversion to thiocyanate using **thiosulphate** administration is an alternative antidote for cyanide poisoning (see this chapter).

3 **Inhibition of metabolism**. An alternative antidotal strategy for situations where a chemical is toxic as a result of metabolism is to block the metabolic transformation. For example, ethylene glycol, often used in antifreeze, is toxic as a result of metabolism first by **alcohol dehydrogenase** and then by other enzymes with the final toxic product being **oxalic acid**. Competitive inhibition of alcohol dehydrogenase with **ethanol** blocks this metabolism and allows the ethylene glycol to be eliminated unchanged. Poisoning with **methanol**, which also involves metabolism by alcohol dehydrogenase, can be treated similarly.

4 **Antidotes acting on a receptor. Morphine** poisoning, which causes respiratory depression, can be treated by blocking the receptor where it acts with the drug **naloxone**. Another example is the treatment of the cholinergic crisis, which occurs as a result of **organophosphate** poisoning, with **atropine**, which antagonizes the effect of the

excess acetylcholine on receptors (see Chapter 8).

5 **Reversal of receptor blockade** or inhibition. Again with poisoning with organophosphates such as **parathion**, the inhibition of the acetylcholinesterase by the metabolite paraoxon can be treated with **pralidoxime** which removes the organophosphate from the enzyme, thereby regenerating it. Another example is the treatment of **carbon monoxide** poisoning with **oxygen**. Because the binding of the carbon monoxide to the haemoglobin is reversible, with a sufficiently high concentration of oxygen this can be displaced. The presence of carbon dioxide also helps to facilitate the dissociation of the carboxyhaemoglobin.

6 Use of **antibodies** or **antibody fragments**. For toxins such as snake venoms, **antivenoms** may be available which specifically bind the protein(s) in the venom. Occasionally antibodies may also be used for the treatment of poisoning with drugs such as **digoxin**.

Summary and learning objectives

There are many chemicals in use in and around the modern home which are potentially poisonous, including potent pesticides, solvents, and strong detergents and acids. A not infrequent culprit of poisoning, often leading to fatalities in the home, is *carbon monoxide* resulting from poor ventilation of stoves, fires and boilers and also found in car exhaust. This gas binds strongly to haemoglobin, thereby competing with and depriving the tissues of oxygen. Symptoms include severe headache, confusion, acidosis, unconsciousness and death from respiratory/cardiac failure. **Ethylene glycol** used in antifreeze may sometimes be ingested, leading to acidosis, kidney and brain damage due to metabolism to toxic aldehydes and acids. A chemical which may be found in the home and also in plants (e.g. Cassava) as well as in factories and laboratories is **cyanide** (usually found as a salt). Cyanide binds to cyto-chrome aa_3 in the mitochondrion, thereby stop-ping the flow of electrons and depleting ATP. Death is usually rapid as a result of cardiac or respiratory failure.

   Alcohol is a ubiquitous but potentially toxic drug which accounts for many cases of liver damage (cirrhosis).

   Solvents and other volatile substances may be inhaled by 'glue-sniffers', leading to uncon-sciousness or sometimes heart failure.

   Treatment of poisoning involves use of eme-tics, absorbants, diuresis and pH manipulation, haemodialysis or haemoperfusion. For some toxic chemicals antidotes exist such as chelating agents, enzyme inhibitors, receptor blockers, antibodies, and agents that increase detoxica-tion or facilitate displacement of toxicants from binding sites.

Questions

Q1. Indicate which of the following are true and which false.
      Ethanol is used as an antidote for the treatment of ethylene glycol poisoning because it:

   a facilitates the excretion of ethylene glycol
   b blocks the metabolism of ethylene glycol

   c increases the detoxication of ethylene glycol
   d chelates ethylene glycol
   e none of the above.

Q2. Carbon monoxide is poisonous because:

   a it binds to cytochrome aa_3 in the mitochondria
   b it binds to haemoglobin
   c it causes respiratory alkalosis
   d it causes a failure of respiration
   e it forms methaemoglobin.

Q3. Indicate which of the following are true with reference to ethylene glycol:

   a it is an alcohol
   b it causes metabolic acidosis
   c it is metabolized to lactic acid
   d it crystallizes in the brain
   e it is metabolized by aldehyde dehy-drogenase.

Q4. Indicate which of the following are true:

   a solvents can cause death by sensitiza-tion of the myocardium
   b alcohol is toxic because it stimulates the central nervous system
   c alcohol is metabolized to formic acid
   d the major target organ for methanol toxicity is the liver
   e large doses of alcohol cause blind-ness
   f high doses of alcohol lower blood sugar.

Q5. Which of the following has been used as an antidote:

   a Lewisite
   b dicobalt edetate
   c thiocyanate
   d N-acetylcysteine
   e pralidoxime.

SHORT ANSWER QUESTION

Q6. Write notes on the various types of general treatment for poisoning.

Bibliography

BACKER, R. C. (1993) Forensic toxicology: a broad overview of general principles, in *General and Applied* Toxicology, Ballantyne, B., Marrs, T. and Turner, P. (Eds), Basingstoke, UK: Macmillan.

Casarett and Doull's Toxicology, The Basic Science of Poisons, C. D. Klaassen (Ed.), 5th edition, 1996, New York: McGraw-Hill. Various chapters.

DREISBACH, R. H. (1983) *Handbook of Poisoning: Diagnosis and Treatment,* 11th edition, Los Altos: C. A. Lange.

ELLENHORN, M. J. and BARCELOUX, D. G. (1988) *Medical Toxicology. Diagnosis and Treatment of Human Poisoning,* New York: Elsevier.

EMSLEY, J. Silent killer in the air we breathe, *The Independent,* 1993.

FLANAGAN, R. J., WIDDOP, B., RAMSEY, J. D. and LOVELAND, M. (1988) Analytical toxicology, *Human Toxicology,* 7, 489–502.

General and Applied Toxicology, Ballantyne, B., Marrs, T. and Syversen, T. L. M. (Eds), 2nd edition, Basingstoke: Macmillan. Various chapters.

GOSSEL, T. A. and BRICKER, J. D. (1994) *Principles of Clinical Toxicology,* 3rd edition, New York: Raven Press.

POLSON, C. J., GREEN, M. A. and LEE, M. R. (1983) *Clinical Toxicology,* London: Pitman.

ROSLING, H. (1988) *Cassava Toxicity and Food Security,* 2nd edition, UNICEF.

SAUL, H. (1994) The debate over the limits, *New Scientist,* 1932, 12–13.

CHAPTER — **12**

Toxicity testing and risk assessment

Chapter outline

In this final chapter you will learn about the testing of chemicals for toxicity and the assessment of risk from chemicals:

- Introduction: evaluation of toxicity

- Human exposure and epidemiology

- Acute toxicity tests

- Sub-chronic toxicity tests

- Chronic toxicity tests

- In vitro toxicity tests

- Risk assessment and interpretation of toxicological data

  - risk assessment

  - hazard identification

  - dose–response assessment

- exposure assessment

- risk characterization

Introduction

In most countries, drugs (including veterinary medicines), food additives and contaminants, industrial chemicals, pesticides and cosmetics, to which humans and other living organisms in the environment may be exposed, have to be evaluated for toxicity. The regulations can vary between countries, however, and it is not within the scope of this book to discuss the regulations in any detail. More information may be gained from the references in the Bibliography. The purpose of Regulatory Toxicology is to ensure that the benefits of chemical substances intended for use by humans outweigh the risks from that use.

Evaluation of toxicity

The toxicity of a chemical can be determined in one of three ways:

a by observing human (or animal or plant) populations exposed to a chemical (**epidemiology**);

b by administering the chemical to animals or plants under controlled conditions and observing the effects (*in vivo*);

c by exposing cells, subcellular fractions or single-celled organisms to the chemical (*in vitro*).

The exposure of humans to chemicals may occur accidentally through the environment, as part of their occupation or intentionally, as with drugs and food additives. Thus, chemical accidents, if thoroughly documented, may provide important information about the toxicity of a chemical in humans. Similarly, exposure of humans to chemicals at work may, if well monitored and recorded, provide evidence of toxicity. Thus, the monitoring of exposure by measuring substances and their metabolites in body fluids and using **biochemical indices** of pathological change may be carried out in humans during potential exposure (see biomarkers, Chapter 4). An example is the monitoring of agricultural workers for exposure to organophosphorus compounds by measuring the degree of inhibition of **cholinesterases** in blood samples. However, acquiring such data is often difficult and is rarely complete or of a good enough standard to be more than additional to animal studies. An exception to this is the experimental administration of industrial chemicals to volunteers. But such chemicals are usually not very toxic and the exposure levels would be very low, only sufficient to determine metabolism and disposition, for exam-

ple. Of particular importance is quantitative exposure data for humans which is often sadly lacking. The development of sensitive and specific biomarkers will improve the acquisition of such data.

Studying particular populations of predatory birds and measuring certain parameters, such as **eggshell thickness** and pesticide level, is an **ecotoxicological** example of testing for toxicity in the field.

Before marketing drugs are first given to a small number of human volunteers and then later to a limited number of patients (**Phase 1 clinical trials**), then to a larger number of patients (**Phase 2 clinical trials**) and then to a large number of patients (**Phase 3 clinical trials**) before being made available to the general public. Both from the clinical trials and the eventual use by the general public, adverse reactions may be detected. Phase 1 trials yield information about metabolism and disposition. Phase 2 and Phase 3 trials yield information about side effects and efficacy.

For human and veterinary medicines in the UK there is a system for reporting adverse reactions to drugs: for human medicines this is the **yellow card system**; for veterinary drugs adverse reactions of both the animal patient and the human user are reported.

Clearly, apart from accidental exposure to high levels and exceptional circumstances where unexpected toxicity occurs, human exposure will normally be to levels that cause little or no toxicity.

Data obtained from human exposure or clinical trials is analysed by epidemiological techniques (although there will be differences between clinical trials that are designed and accidental or occupational exposure). Typically, effects observed will be compared to those in control subjects with the objective of determining if there is an association between exposure to the chemical and a disease or adverse effect.

There are four types of epidemiological study:

a **Cohort studies** in which individuals exposed to the chemical of interest are followed over time *prospectively*.

b **Case-control studies** in which individuals who have been exposed and may have developed a disease are compared *retrospectively* with similar control subjects who have no disease.

c **Cross-sectional studies** in which the prevalence of a disease in an exposed group is studied.

d **Ecological studies** where the incidence of a disease in one geographical area (where there may be hazardous chemical exposure) is compared with the incidence in another area without the hazardous chemical.

For accidental, unintentional exposure the analysis is normally *retrospective* and will be a 'case-control study'. The control population will be human subjects chosen to be as similar as possible for age, sex and other parameters. This type of design would be used for studying the relationship between exposure to a volatile chemical in the workplace and lung cancer, for example. Of course there will be a prevalence of lung cancer in the controls but the intention is to discover if the prevalence is higher in those exposed to the chemical. Another example is of drugs already in use in the general population where adverse drug reactions (**ADRs**) in patients are reported by clinicians. For this type of design the data can be represented as an **odds ratio**[*] which is an estimate of relative risk.

The other type of design is *prospective* (known as a cohort study) and is used in clinical trials of drugs. Controls are subjects selected out of the patient population and have the disease

for which the drug is prescribed. The controls receive an inactive '**placebo**'.

Epidemiological data can be analysed in various ways to give measures of effect. The data can be represented as an *odds ratio*[*] which is the ratio of the risk of disease in an exposed group compared to a control group. The **relative risk** is determined as the ratio of the occurrence of the disease in the exposed to the unexposed population. The **absolute excess risk** is an alternative quantitative measure[#].

When setting up epidemiological studies and when assessing their significance it is important to be aware of confounding factors such as bias and the need for proper controls.

For further details on epidemiology the reader is referred to the bibliography.

Although human data from epidemiological studies is useful, the majority of data on the toxicity of chemicals is gained from experimental studies in animals. The data so acquired is used for the risk assessment and safety evaluation of drugs prior to human exposure, for food additives before use and for industrial and environmental chemicals. In the case of drugs this information is essential before the drug can be administered to patients and for food additives and other chemicals it is required in order to set a No Observed Adverse Effect Level (**NOAEL**, see this chapter).

Because animal tests can be carefully controlled with the doses known exactly, the qual-

---

[*] Calculated as: $A \times B/C \times D$

A = no. of cases of disease in exposed population; B = no. of unexposed controls without disease; C = no. of exposed subjects without disease; D = no. of unexposed controls with disease.

[#] Relative risk calculated as: A/B where A = no. of cases of disease in total exposed group per unit of population; B = no. of cases of disease in total non-exposed control group per unit of population.

Absolute excess risk calculated as: no. of cases of disease per unit of exposed population minus no. of cases of disease per unit of unexposed population.

ity of the data is generally good. The number of animals used should be enough to allow statistical significance to be demonstrated. Humane conditions and proper treatment of animals is essential for scientific as well as ethical reasons as this helps to ensure that the data is reliable and robust. The problem of extrapolation between animal species and humans always has to be considered but past data as well as theoretical considerations indicate that in the majority of cases toxic effects occurring in animals will also occur in humans.

The conduct of the animal toxicity tests required depend partly on the type of substance and its expected use and also on the regulations of the particular country. The amount of data necessary also depends on the end use of the substance. For instance, industrial chemicals produced in small quantities may only require minimal toxicity data whereas drugs to be administered to humans require extensive toxicological testing. Pesticides may have to be tested on many different types of animal and plant in the environment and examined for their persistence and behaviour in food chains. The stability of such substances in particular environments is also of importance. Consequently, ecotoxicology involves more extensive residue analysis than does drug toxicology. However, for veterinary medicines, determination of residues in food for human consumption is required.

The species selected will depend partly on the type of toxicity test, data available and also ethical and financial considerations. For example, although the old world monkey, being generally the most similar to humans, might be the desirable species to use for a particular toxicity evaluation, both cost and ethical reasons will often rule this out. The most common species used are rats and mice for reasons of size, accumulated knowledge of these species and cost. Currently, mice have the advantage in being available as **genetically modified** varieties. To show and evaluate some types of toxic effect a particular species might be required.

For veterinary drugs or environmental pollutants the target species will normally be used. Normally young adult animals of both sexes will be used. The exposure level of the chemical used will ideally span both non-toxic and maximally toxic doses.

Examples of pertinent questions which should be asked *before* any toxicity evaluation are:

1 is it a **novel compound** or has it been in use for some time?

2 is it to be **released into the environment**?

3 is it to be **added to human food**?

4 is it to be given as a **single dose** or repeatedly?

5 at what **dosage level** is it to be administered?

6 what **age group** will be exposed?

7 are **pregnant women** or women of childbearing age likely to be exposed?

Toxicity may be an *intrinsic* property of a molecule which results from interaction with a particular biological system. Consequently, a knowledge of the **physico-chemical properties** of that molecule may help the toxicologist to understand the toxicity or potential toxicity and to predict the likely disposition and metabolism. Indeed, we have seen several examples in this book of the importance of physico-chemical principles in toxicology. **Structure–activity relationships** are beginning to be used in toxicology as they are in pharmacology, especially in the field of chemical mutagenesis/carcinogenesis. This initial knowledge from preliminary studies may also influence the course of the subsequent toxicity tests especially if there are similarities with other compounds of known toxicity. Hence, the solubility, partition coefficient, melting or boiling point, vapour pressure and purity are important parameters. For example, an industrial chemical which is a very volatile liquid (i.e. with a high vapour pressure) should at least be tested for toxicity by inhalation and possibly by skin application.

As well as physico-chemical considerations there are also biological considerations and the following are the major ones:

1 the most appropriate **species** to study,

2 the **sex** of the animals used,

3 the use of **inbred** or **outbred** strains,

4 **housing**,

5 **diet**,

6 animal **health**,

7 **metabolic similarity to man**,

8 the **route of administration**,

9 **duration** of the toxicity study,

10 the **numbers** of animals used,

11 **vehicle**.

The route of administration and vehicle will depend on the expected end use or, if a drug for example, on the means of administration. The parameters to be measured may also be dependent on the particular study. For example, metabolic studies can be combined with a toxicity study and plasma levels measured as well as urinary metabolites identified and clinical chemical parameters studied. The biochemical and pathological measurements to be made will also be decided before the study is started.

Initial toxicity studies will usually be carried out to determine the *approximate range of toxic dosage*. For a drug this may already be known from pharmacological studies but for an industrial chemical, for instance, nothing

may be known of its biological activity. Consequently, the initial range-finding studies may utilize dosage on a logarithmic scale or half-log scale. These initial studies are important if large numbers of animals are not to be wasted in later studies. The initial tests will also involve *observation* of the animals in order to gain insight into the possible toxic effects.

Once the approximate toxic dosage range is known then various detailed toxicity studies can be carried out. These will be followed by various other toxicity tests, usually including the following: **acute, sub-chronic (28- or 90-day), chronic (lifetime), mutagenicity, carcinogenicity, teratogenicity, reproductive studies** and *in vitro* **tests**. For some compounds there may also be other types of toxicity test such as **irritancy** and **skin sensitization** studies.

There are different requirements for drugs, food additives and contaminants, industrial chemicals, cosmetics and pesticides because of the different circumstances of exposure. Chemicals which are to be used in the environment, such as pesticides and industrial chemicals which might be accidently released into the environment, will also undergo **ecotoxicity** tests. These will include tests with invertebrates such as *Daphnia*, **earthworms, fish, phytoplankton** and **higher plants**.

Acute toxicity tests

Acute toxicity tests are those designed to determine the effects which occur within a short period after dosing. These tests can determine a **dose–response relationship** and the **LD_{50} value** if required. The exact conduct of toxicity studies will vary depending on the compound, its eventual use and the particular regulations to be satisfied. Usually at least four dosages are used which may be in *logarithmic progression* especially if no range-finding studies have been done. However, the traditional LD_{50} determination is now no longer required by most regulatory authorities. (For more information on this test see the publications in the Bibliography.) Recently an *alternative* to this test which attempts to find the approximate toxic dosage but uses far *fewer animals* has been suggested by the **British Toxicology Society**. In this procedure a small number of animals, such as five of each sex, are exposed to the chemical under test at a dosage level of 5 mg kg^{-1} (for example) and observed for **signs of toxicity**. If 90 per cent or more of the animals survive without signs of toxicity then a larger dosage, such as 50 mg kg^{-1} is employed. If again 90 per cent or more survive without signs of toxicity then the chemical is termed unclassified. Depending on the dosage required for toxicity to be evident then the chemical can be classified as shown in Table 12.1.

The information to be gained from an acute toxicity test is the nature of the dose–response relationship and observations on the toxic effects and time to death, if any of the animals die. It is important that the dosage range used is wide enough for toxic effects to be manifested at the highest dosages used unless this would require doses that were unrealistic in relation to the expected dose or exposure. The dosage range and the method of administration will be influenced by the expected or intended route of administration and likely dosage or exposure concentration.

At the end of the toxicity test the surviving animals are killed and undergo a **post-mortem** with a **pathological examination** of tissues. Animals dying during the study should also undergo a post-mortem.

Sub-chronic toxicity tests

Following acute toxicity tests, sub-chronic toxicity tests are usually carried out. These involve exposing the animals to the substance under test for a prolonged period, usually 28 or 90 days. The exposure is frequent and usually **daily**. These tests provide information on the **target organs** affected by the compound and the major toxic effects. Toxic effects which have a slow onset can be detected and *reversible* and *adaptive* responses may become apparent during the test. Measurements of **levels** of the compound in **blood** and **tissues** can be made and this information correlated with any toxic effects seen. At the end of the study pathological examination is carried out

TABLE 12.1 *Investigation of acute oral toxicity and estimation of maximum non-lethal oral dosage for classification purposes*

Test dosage	Result	Action/classification
5 mg kg^{-1}	<90% survival	*Very toxic*
	>90% survival but toxicity	*Toxic*
	>90% survival no toxicity	Retest at 50 mg kg^{-1}
50 mg kg^{-1}	<90% survival	*Toxic*; test / retest at 5 mg kg^{-1}
	>90% survival but toxicity	*Harmful*
	>90% survival no toxicity	Retest at 500 mg kg^{-1}
500 mg kg^{-1}	<90% survival or toxicity	*Harmful*; test /retest at 50 mg kg^{-1}
	>90% survival no toxicity	*Unclassified*

This table has been adapted from M. J. van den Heuvel *et al., Human Toxicology,* **6**, 279, 1987.

and during the study **clinical chemical measurements** should indicate the development of any pathological lesions. The data derived from sub-chronic toxicity studies also help in the *design* of chronic toxicity studies. Attempts are usually made in sub-chronic toxicity studies to identify a **no-observed effect level**, taking data from other tests into consideration.

Chronic toxicity tests

These tests involve exposure of animals to the compounds of interest for at least 12 months to 2 years in rodents (about 50 per cent lifespan) and 6–12 months in non-rodents. Chronic toxicity tests may be combined with *in vivo* carcinogenicity tests, in which case the exposure of rodents will be lifetime, and satellite groups may be used for interim chronic toxicity information. There is currently discussion in the International Committee on Harmonisation as to whether chronic toxicity tests need to be as long as 2 years or whether shorter times will yield as much information. As with sub-chronic toxicity tests the chronic toxicity test will *terminate* with a **pathological examination** and there may also be **clinical chemical measurements** made throughout at intervals. These clinical chemical measurements can indicate the development of pathological changes which can then be detected at post-mortem. Changes in other simple measurements such as **body weight** and **food** and **water intake** may also indicate adverse effects. Chronic toxicity studies are important for drugs administered over *long periods of time*, for food additives to which we may be exposed for our *whole lifetimes* and for environmental and industrial chemicals where we may be exposed to *low levels* for *long periods*.

For all three types of toxicity test, selection of dosages, species, strain of animal, route of exposure, parameters measured and many other considerations are vitally important. These considerations will clearly be influenced by the particular type of chemical, expected circumstances of exposure and the regulations of the countries in which the substance is to be used. For details of these toxicity tests the reader is referred to the texts given in the Bibliography.

The requirements of the New Substances Notification Scheme in the EU serve to illustrate the range of physico-chemical, toxicological and ecotoxicological studies that may be required. Under these regulations the amount of testing required depends upon the amount of the substance produced but an indication of the requirements is shown in Table 12.2. (For further information see Fairhurst, S., chapter 67, and Auer, C. M. and Fielder, R. J., chapter 72, in Ballantyne, Marrs and Syversen, 1999 in Bibliography). In addition, teratology, fertility, further subchronic, carcinogenicity and chronic toxicity studies may be required *depending on the amount* of the compound produced and the results of other tests. It may also be necessary to repeat some of the studies already carried out but using alternative routes of administration or a different species of animal for instance. Similarly **ecotoxicology** studies may also need to be increased to include *prolonged* toxicity studies in *Daphnia* and fish, effects on higher plants and determination of **bioaccumulation** in fish and possibly other species. The tests described are the basic ones required and serve to illustrate the principles involved. However, other tests will also be required such as teratogenicity and other reproductive studies, carcinogenicity, mutagenicity, irritancy and skin sensitization.

Reproductive studies determine the effect of the compound on the *reproductive process*. Thus, **teratogenicity tests** examine the effect

TABLE 12.2 *The type of information required (including toxicity) for a new chemical substance under the EU New Substances Notification Scheme*

Identity	Toxicology studies
name / trade name	acute toxicity (oral / inhalation / cutaneous)
formulae (empirical / structural)	skin and eye irritancy
composition	skin sensitization
methods of detection / determination	subacute toxicity (28 days)
	mutagenicity (bacterial and non-bacterial)
Uses and Precautions	**Ecotoxicological studies**
proposed uses	toxicity to fish
estimated production / importation	toxicity to *Daphnia*
handling / storage / transport methods and precautions	degradation data (BOD, BOD / COD)
emergency measures	
Physico-chemical properties	**Possibility of rendering substances harmless**
melting point	for industry
boiling point	for public
relative density	declaration concerning the possibility of unfavourable effects
vapour pressure	proposed classification and labelling
surface tension	proposals for any recommended precautions for safe use
water solubility	
fat solubility	
partition coefficient (octanol / water)	
flash point	
flammability	
explosive properties	
auto-flammability	
oxidizing properties	

Further information from Fairhurst, S., chapter 67, and Auer, C. M. and Fielder, R. J., chapter 72, in Ballantyne, Marrs and Syversen, 1999, see Bibliography.

of the compound on the development of the embryo and foetus. These may be detected as gross anatomical *abnormalities* in the newborn animal or may be more subtle effects such as changes in behaviour. The effect of the compound on the **fertility** of both male and female animals may also be determined in reproductive toxicity tests. Data from other tests may also be relevant, such as pathological evidence of testicular damage which might additionally be detected as a decrease in male fertility.

Mutagenicity tests determine whether the compound has potential to cause **genetic damage** and so induce a mutation in germ cells and somatic cells. Such tests indicate whether a compound may have the potential to induce cancers. Mutagenicity tests are carried out in **bacteria** and **cultured mammalian cells**

in vitro. *In vivo* assays include the **micro-nucleus test** and the **dominant lethal assay** (see Bibliography for details).

Carcinogenicity tests may also be required, especially if the mutagenicity tests are positive. The compound is given for the lifetime of the animal, administered either in the drinking water or diet. The appearance of tumours at post-mortem or perhaps before the animal dies are detected from histopathological studies of sections of tissues from the major organs.

Irritancy and **skin sensitization tests** may also be required, especially for industrial chemicals and pesticides. **Irritancy tests** are sometimes carried out on rabbit skin or eyes. The **skin sensitization test** is normally carried out in the guinea pig and a positive result indicates that the compound has the potential to cause contact dermatitis in humans. Some compounds may also cause **pulmonary sensitization** but there is no reliable animal model for this effect. Consideration of the toxicity data may suggest that further studies be carried out, such as an investigation to show that an effect is peculiar to a particular species and therefore not relevant to man.

Toxicity tests are normally either carried out by the company producing the compound or a **contract research laboratory** or a combination of both. The conduct of the toxicity and eco-toxicity studies should conform to certain guidelines, such as those issued by the **Organisation for Economic Cooperation and Development (OECD)**. These guidelines are often enshrined in national regulatory requirements such as those in the UK and USA. Toxicity tests also now must be carried out in compliance with a system known as **Good Laboratory Practice (GLP)**, which governs every aspect of the conduct of studies including the reporting of results. This system was introduced to ensure that toxicity tests are competently carried out and that data is not fabricated, following a notorious situation which arose in the USA.

As well as the requirements of regulatory agencies, toxicity data may also have other uses. Indeed, the data may be life saving in cases of human and animal poisoning. For example, animal studies on **cyanide toxicity** provided data which was useful in the **treatment of poisoning** with cyanide. The *absence* of any toxicity data on **methylisocyanate** probably hampered the efforts of rescue workers and clinicians at **Bhopal** in India after the massive disaster where methylisocyanate leaked from a chemical plant there. Basic studies on **paracetamol toxicity** led directly to the use of an **antidote** which has proved extremely successful and life saving. Attempts to understand the mechanisms underlying the toxicity of compounds will allow better prediction of toxicity and also better design of tests to discover toxic potential.

Testing in vitro

It has become necessary to question the use of *in vivo* safety evaluation studies because of the pressure from society to reduce the use of live animals in medical research. Consequently, there has been an increase in the exploration and use of various *in vitro* systems in toxicity testing. The current philosophy is embodied in the concept of the **three R's**: **replacement**, **reduction** and **refinement**. Thus, if possible, live animals should be *replaced* with alternatives. If this is not possible then measures should be adopted to *reduce* the numbers used. Finally, research workers should also *refine* the methods used to ensure greater animal welfare and reduction in distress and improve the quality of the data derived, if possible.

In some areas the use of *in vitro* systems has been successful. For example the use of *in vitro* tests for the detection of genotoxicity is now well established. These tests include the well known **Ames test** which relies on detecting mutations in **bacteria** (*Salmonella typhimurium*). These are useful early screens for detecting potential toxicity, in particular genotoxicity, which may lead to the production of tumours in whole animals.

Other microorganisms such as *E. coli* bacteria and **yeast** may be used. Mammalian cells are also used for tests for genotoxicity, typically **mouse lymphoma** or **Chinese hamster ovary** cell lines. Human lymphocytes can also be used for the detection of chromosomal damage. Fruit flies are sometimes used for specific tests such as the detection of sex-linked recessive lethal mutations. However, the correlation between a positive result for mutagenicity in tests such as the bacterial test and carcinogenicity in an animal is not 100 per cent. That is, known animal carcinogens are not universally mutagenic in the bacterial tests and *vice versa* some mutagenic chemicals are not carcinogenic in animals. Therefore although *in vitro* bacterial tests may be used to screen out potential genotoxic carcinogens, those compounds which are not apparently mutagenic may still have to be tested for carcinogenicity *in vivo*.

One area where *in vitro* tests have been successful is in the testing of **cosmetics**. The use of skin cells and simpler *in vitro* systems has allowed the cosmetic industry to dramatically reduce the use of *in vivo* testing of substances for irritancy, for example. However, human skin is generally more readily available than other human tissues and is also more readily utilized in *in vitro* systems.

Apart from bacterial mutagenicity tests and other such tests using single-celled organisms and skin testing, other *in vitro* systems are still not yet widely used as alternatives to *in vivo*

experiments. However, progress is being made and recently an *in vitro* alternative to the *in vivo* test for **allergenicity/sensitization** was developed. However, currently many of these tests do not stand alone and require additional data to be gathered *in vivo*. For example, although a bacterial mutagenicity test might indicate a chemical is a potential genotoxic carcinogen, actual carcinogenicity can only be demonstrated in an animal *in vivo*. A positive result in the bacterial test might be sufficient to stop development of a drug but with other compounds such as industrial chemicals which may already be in use, an indication of the actual carcinogenicity may be needed. Similarly, with a cosmetic in development, a positive result in an *in vitro* test might be sufficient to stop development but with other chemicals a more definitive answer may be needed.

One of the *in vitro* systems most used is the **isolated liver cell**. These may be primary liver cells derived from animal or human liver or alternatively cell lines, such as **HepG2** cells, derived from liver tumours.

Unfortunately there are a number of problems with many of the *in vitro* systems currently in use which makes the use of such systems for prediction and risk assessment difficult. Thus, primary cells may show poor viability in medium to long-term experiments and this may limit their usefulness to short-term exposure. There are also major biochemical changes which occur with time in primary cells, starting from almost the moment of preparation of the tissue. Changes, such as in the level and proportions of isozymes of **cytochrome P450** which occur over the first 24 hours after isolation for instance will influence the toxicity of chemicals in those cells if metabolic activation is a factor.

An alternative *in vitro* system is the use of cell lines, immortal cells which will continue to grow and can be frozen and used when needed. These cells are not, however, the same as those in normal tissue and are often derived from tumours.

When comparisons have been made with *in vivo* data, in many cases the *in vitro* system reacts differently to the tissue in the animal *in vivo*. This difference may be qualitative or quantitative. Therefore, although *in vitro* systems are used and are especially useful for mechanistic studies, the data generated from them has to be viewed with caution. This is particularly the case if the data is being used as part of a risk assessment. Such *in vitro* data may underestimate the toxicity *in vivo*.

Thus, it is not yet possible to replace all animal experiments with *in vitro* systems even though considerable progress has been made. *In vitro* systems are particularly useful, however, for screening out toxic compounds which might otherwise be developed, for mechanistic studies and for comparing different compounds within a group of analogues for example.

Risk assessment and interpretation of toxicological data

At least *65 000 chemicals* are currently produced in the USA with 500–1000 new chemicals added each year. In the past, perhaps chemicals were too readily produced and used without due care and attention. **Rachel Carson** in her book, *Silent Spring* showed the risks of such actions. The general public is now very suspicious of all chemicals and there is perhaps an exaggerated fear of poisoning from chemicals in the environment and a belief that all chemicals are hazardous. Regulation has been introduced in many countries in response to this public fear and pressure. Clearly regulation is

necessary, but where possible guidelines should be issued rather than strict rules for the assessment of every case in the same way. A major problem with toxicological data is the assessment of **hazards** and the subsequent calculation of **risks** and estimation of **risk versus benefit**.

RISK ASSESSMENT

Risk is a mathematical concept which refers to the likelihood of undesirable effects resulting from exposure to a chemical.

Risk may be defined as the probability that a hazard will cause an adverse effect under specific exposure conditions.

Risk may also be defined in the following way: Risk = hazard × exposure.

Hazard may be defined as the intrinsic capability of a substance to cause an adverse effect.

Conversely, safety may be defined as 'the practical certainty that adverse effects will not occur when the substance is used in the manner and quantity proposed for its use'.

As exposure increases so does the probability of harm and therefore a reduction in exposure reduces the risk.

Risk assessment would be carried out on chemicals for the following reasons:

a the chemical is likely to be a **hazard** to humans in the environment;

b the likelihood of **persistence** of the chemical in the environment and bioaccumulation;

c the likelihood that **sensitive human** and **ecological** populations may be exposed to significant levels;

d indication of hazard to **human** health;

e   likelihood of **exposure** via use or production.

Risk assessment is the process whereby hazard, exposure and risk are determined. An underlying concept in risk assessment relies on the statement by Paracelsus (see Chapter 1), and so for many, although not all chemicals, there will be a dose–effect relationship. Therefore the corrollary is that there should be a safe dose. Consequently, it should be possible to determine a level of exposure that is without appreciable risk to human health or the ecosystem. Risk assessment is a scientific process. The next stages are risk benefit analysis and risk management that require a different type of approach.

Risk management is a process of considering alternative policies and choosing the most appropriate course of regulatory action based on the results of risk assessment and social, economic and political considerations.

Risk assessment is the process whereby the nature and magnitude of the risk is determined. It requires four steps:

i   **Hazard identification**. This is the evaluation of the toxic effects of the chemical in question.

ii   Demonstration of a **dose–response** or dose–effect relationship. Evaluation of the causal relationship between the exposure to the hazard and an adverse effect in individuals or populations, respectively.

iii **Exposure assessment**. Determination of the level, frequency and duration of exposure of humans to the hazardous substance.

iv   **Risk characterization**. Estimation of the incidence of adverse effects under the various conditions of human exposure.

Considering each of these in turn:

Hazard identification

This is the evaluation of the *potential* of a chemical to cause toxicity. The data used is normally derived from:

a   **human epidemiology**

b   **animal toxicity studies**

c   *in vivo* and *in vitro* **mechanistic** or other **studies**.

A chemical may constitute a number of hazards of different severity. However, the *primary hazard* will be the one used for the subsequent stages of the risk assessment process. For example, a chemical may cause reversible liver toxicity at high doses but cause tumours in the skin at lower doses. The carcinogenicity is clearly the hazard of concern.

Although human data is ideal, reliable data from humans is not often available and must be supplemented with other data in order to define a dose–response relationship. However, epidemiological data may at least indicate that a **causal relationship** exists between exposure to the chemical and an effect in humans. Therefore, in practice, animal toxicity data is normally required. This will be generated by toxicity studies that are controlled and that generate histopathological, clinical chemical and biochemical data (see Chapter 4 and this chapter). Of course, the differences between humans and other species must always be recognized and taken into account (see below). It may be possible to use *in vitro* data both from human cells and tissues as well as those from other animals to supplement the epidemiological and animal *in vivo* toxicity data. However, at present such data cannot *replace* experimental animal or human epidemiological data. The predictive use of structure activity relationships is also possible and an approach which is becoming increasingly important.

Dose–response assessment

This stage quantitates the hazards already identified and estimates the relationship between the dose and the adverse effect in humans. However, this requires extrapolation from possibly high, experimental doses used in animals to levels likely to be encountered by humans.

The extrapolation from high to low doses will depend on the type of primary toxic effect. If this is a carcinogenic effect then a **threshold** normally cannot be assumed and a mathematical model is used to estimate the risk at low doses. If the primary toxic effect is non-carcinogenic then it will normally be assumed that a threshold exists.

Risk assessment of carcinogens is a two-step process involving, firstly, a qualitative assessment of the data from the hazard identification stage (see above) and, secondly, a quantitation of the risk for definitive or probable human carcinogens.

The first stage uses either the EPA or IARC classification system which are very similar. The IARC system is shown below.

IARC classification of chemicals in relation to carcinogenicity:

Group 1 *The agent is carcinogenic to humans.* This category is used when there is sufficient evidence of carcinogenicity in humans (e.g. aflatoxin, benzene, arsenic, tobacco smoke).

Group 2A *The agent is probably carcinogenic in humans.* This category is used when there is limited evidence of carcinogenicity in humans but convincing evidence of carcinogenicity in experimental animals (e.g. acrylonitrile, cadmium, benzo[a]pyrene).

Group 2B *The agent is possibly carcinogenic in humans.* This category is used when there is only limited evidence of carcinogenicity in humans and less than convincing evidence of carcinogenicity in experimental animals (e.g. carbon tetrachloride, urethane, hexachlorobenzene).

Group 3 *The agent is not classifiable as to its carcinogenicity.* This is used when the evidence for carcinogenicity of the agent in humans and experimental animals is inadequate (e.g. aniline, dieldrin, maneb).

Group 4 *The agent is probably not carcinogenic in humans.* This is used when the agent has not been found to induce cancer in either experimental animals or humans despite thorough testing (e.g. Caprolactam).

For group 1 the data should show a causal relationship between exposure and cancer in humans. For chemicals classified as group 1 or 2A the second stage is a quantitative risk assessment. The classification may change for a chemical when more information becomes available.

There are several models that can be used and these range from ultraconservative to least conservative:

a   the **one-hit model**. This is ultra-conservative as it assumes that cancer involves only one stage and a single molecular event is sufficient to induce a cellular transformation.

b   The **linearized Multistage Model** (used by the EPA). This determines the cancer slope factor that can be used to predict cancer risk at a specific dose. It assumes a linear extrapolation to a zero dose threshold (see Figure 1.7). This factor is an estimate (expressed in mg/kg/day) of the probability that an individual will develop cancer if exposed to the chemical for 70 years.

c   The **multi-hit model**, which assumes several interactions are necessary for transformation of a normal to a cancerous cell.

d **Probit model**. This assumes a log normal distribution for tolerance in the exposed population.

Another model that is increasingly being used is the **physiologically based pharmacokinetic model**. This utilizes data on the absorption, distribution, metabolism, tissue sequestration, kinetics, elimination and mechanism to determine the target dose used for the extrapolation but it requires extensive data.

The cancer risk values that these models generate are of course very different. For example for the chemical **chlordane**, the lifetime risk for one cancer death in one million people ranges from 0.03 $\mu g\,l^{-1}$ of drinking water for the one-hit model, 0.07 $\mu g\,l^{-1}$ from the linearized multi-stage model to 50 $\mu g\,l^{-1}$ for the probit model.

The results from **animal carcinogenicity testing** studies are particularly hard to assess as it is necessary but difficult to show an *increased frequency* of tumours in a small population such as those used in animal cancer studies, in which there may already be a significant incidence of some types of tumours. There is a practical, statistical limit which determines the incidence or frequency of occurrence of a cancer which can be detected. For example, using 1000 animals it is necessary for more than five animals to be affected by cancer for the effect to be detected at the 99 per cent confidence level; but an incidence of five cases in 1000 test animals if extrapolated to man would translate into over *1 million cases* of cancer in a population the size of that of the US. To use even larger numbers of animals would be impractical, extremely expensive, and challenged on ethical (animal rights) grounds. So assessing cancer risk from carcinogenicity studies is very difficult and those conducting and assessing the tests tend to err on the side of caution. One way around the dilemma of low incidence is to *increase the doses* used in the

animal tests on the assumption that the dose-response is linear and so extrapolation backwards is possible. This has given rise to various models but estimates from these models vary; the precision of the mathematical model is largely irrelevant if the quality of the original toxicological data is poor. There may be large margins of error and uncertainty. Unfortunately the public may take the exposure limits and similar data issued at face value or alternately disbelieve them completely. Consequently, doses close to the **Maximum Tolerated Dose (MTD)** are used in carcinogenicity testing despite the problems of **dose-dependent metabolism**, **dose-dependent kinetics**, and the possibility of other pathological effects influencing the carcinogenicity. This approach is contentious, however, as carcinogens may show dose-dependent metabolism and with weak or equivocal carcinogens such as **saccharin** (see Chapter 7) and especially non-genotoxic carcinogens this may be crucial to the interpretation of the carcinogenicity data. That is, large doses of a compound may be metabolized in a quantitatively or qualitatively different manner to that of the expected dose or exposure level. Consequently, a compound may only be carcinogenic under those extreme dosing conditions. For example, the industrial chemical **hydrazine** is a *weak* carcinogen after high exposure or dose levels. It also causes **DNA methylation**, a *possibly* mutagenic event which might lead to cancer but this methylation only occurs after *large*, hepatotoxic doses. The implications of this are that the acute toxic effect is in some way involved in the DNA methylation and that also the acute effect is necessary for the development of the cancer. For non-carcinogens where the dose response shows a threshold, a dose can be determined at which there is no adverse effect, the **No Adverse Effect Level (NOAEL)** (see Figure 1.7). The effect will be one that is likely to occur in humans and that is the most sensitive toxic effect observed. If a NOAEL cannot be determined (if the data is insufficiently robust) then the **Lowest Adverse Effect Level (LOAEL)** is determined.

Exposure assessment

Exposure to a chemical converts it from being a hazard into a risk. Thus determination of exposure is crucial to the whole process of risk assessment. This involves evaluation of the source of the exposure, the routes by which humans are exposed and the level of exposure.

Of course in some situations of exposure to chemicals, such as around waste disposal areas or chemical factories, exposure is to a mixture of possibly many different chemicals. These may interact in a variety of ways (e.g. additivity, synergism, antagonism, potentiation, see Chapter 1). Exposure may be by more than one route (inhalation, skin contact, ingestion) and different types of organism may be exposed (human, animal, adult, infant). Therefore the real life situation of exposure to chemicals in the workplace or environment can be immensely complex when these factors are taken into account. Risk assessment requires a consideration of these.

Actual exposure levels may not always be known and therefore models may have to be used that utilize knowledge of air dispersion or ground water movements.

The **physico-chemical characteristics** of the chemical in question (i.e. lipid solubility, water solubility, vapour pressure, etc.) also will be important information.

However, the risk assessment process is more reliable if there is an indication of actual exposures for both the experimental animals and humans that have provided the data on which it is based. The exposure assessment may use **biomarkers** to improve the process (see below).

Risk characterization

The final stage involves integration of the results of the preceding stages to get a probability of the occurrence of the adverse effect in humans exposed to the chemical. The biological, statistical and other uncertainties will have to be taken into account.

For carcinogens the risk is expressed in terms of increased risk of developing a cancer (e.g. 1 in 10^6). This is calculated from the **cancer slope factor** and the 70-year average daily intake in mg/kg/day.

From the NOAEL (or LOAEL if there is no reliable NOAEL) various parameters can be determined.

For food additives this is normally the **Acceptable Daily Intake (ADI)** (or the **Reference Dose, Rfd,** used by the Environmental Protection Agency in the USA). The ADI is the amount of chemical to which a person can be exposed for a lifetime without suffering harmful effects. The determination of these intake values requires the use of a safety or uncertainty factor. The RfD includes an additional safety factor (modifying factor, see below). For food contaminants the parameter is the **Tolerable Daily Intake (TDI)**. The TDI is an estimate of the daily intake of the chemical that can occur over a lifetime without appreciable health risk. Daily food consumption for a particular type of food will be used for this calculation.

Food may also contain veterinary drug residues and the pesticide residues for which ADIs may be calculated.

Chemicals in water and air also have to be assessed for risk and guidelines set where appropriate. Thus there are air quality/pollution guidelines set by the World Health Organisation (WHO). Air pollutants may have acute irritant effects or chronic effects or both. The guidance values give levels combined with exposure times at which no adverse effects would be expected. The guidance values are determined from the NOAEL (or LOAEL).

Similarly there are drinking water guidance values for a number of chemicals. For drinking water contaminants as with food contaminants a Tolerable Daily Intake can be established from the NOAEL and appropriate safety factors. The guidance value is determined from the TDI and known daily intake of water by a standard adult of 60 kg weight drinking the water for 70 years. As with air pollutants, carcinogenic, non-threshold chemicals will be considered differently to non-carcinogenic chemicals where there is considered to be no threshold.

In the case of carcinogens a **Virtually Safe Dose (VSD)** may be determined.

The modifying or safety factors are as follows:

10× for **human variability (intra species)**;
10× for **extrapolation** from animals to humans (**interspecies variability**);
10× **if less than chronic doses** have been used;
10× **if** the **LOAEL** rather than the NOAEL is used;
0.1–10× modifying factor. This is only used for determination of the RfD (EPA).

These **uncertainty factors** are combined and divided into the NOAEL (or LOAEL) to give the ADI (or RfD) or TDI. The modifying factor allows for judgement on the quality of the scientific data.

Thus:

$$TDI = NOAEL/Uncertainty\ factor(s)$$

$$ADI = NOAEL/Uncertainty\ factor(s)$$

Often an uncertainty factor of 100 is applied to account for human variability and for differences between humans and the animals used in the toxicity studies.

This approach can be applied to both chronic and shorter term (e.g. developmental) toxicity and similar methods may be used to derive permissible exposure levels for acute and short-term exposure. Clearly the toxicity data used would be derived from studies of appropriate length. For **occupational exposure** to chemicals as opposed to environmental exposure other parameters such as **Threshold Limit Values (or Maximum Exposure Limits)** are determined in a similar way and are based on exposure for an eight-hour working day.

Doses are normally either expressed on a body weight or body surface area basis and are then extrapolated to a different species. This assumes similar sensitivity per unit body weight or surface area. Thus in the risk assessment process for non-carcinogens the actual exposure level is compared with the ADI or other equivalent parameter for example. Exposure to multiple chemicals will be assumed to be additive.

Extrapolation *between species* is also a problem in risk assessment and the interpretation of toxicological data. For example, one question that arises is 'which species is the extrapolation to be made from, the most sensitive or the one which in terms of response or disposition of the compound is the most similar to man?' The species or strain used in a particular carcinogenicity study may have a high natural incidence of a specific type or types of tumour. The assessment of the significance of an increase in the incidence of this tumour and its relevance to man can pose particular problems. Therefore, risk assessment from carcinogenicity is fraught with difficulties, possibly more than any other type of toxic effect.

For acute toxic effects the dose response is often clear cut and allows a **NOAEL** to be estimated. However, the biology of the toxicity study must always be taken into account and a too exaggerated reliance on statistics must be avoided. Because of the problems of interspecies extrapolation and interpretation of low incidences of tumours, risk assessment may give rise to widely disparate quantitative values. For example, for **saccharin** the expected number of **bladder cancer** cases in the USA over a 70-year period due to daily exposure to 120 mg was *estimated* as between 0.22 and 1.144×10^6! Therefore, in the risk assessment of a particular compound other factors become important such as the *likely* and *reasonable* human exposure but in the USA the strict rules of the **Delaney clause** make this difficult (see Glossary for definition of Delaney Clause).

THE USE OF BIOMARKERS IN RISK ASSESSMENT

Biomarkers are used at several stages in the risk assessment process. Biomarkers of exposure are important in risk assessment as an indication of the ***internal* dose** is necessary for the proper description of the dose–response relationship. Similarly, biomarkers of response are necessary for determination of the NOAEL and the dose–response relationship. Biomarkers of susceptibility may be important for determining specially sensitive groups for estimating an uncertainty factor. Biomarkers allow the crucial link between the response and exposure to be established.

The incidence of a toxic effect may be measured under precise laboratory conditions but extrapolation to a real life situation to give an estimate of risk involves many *assumptions* and gives rise to *uncertainties*. The risk assessor has to decide which are plausible answers to questions when in reality there are either no scientific answers or these answers are obscure.

For a new chemical substance human data is not available and toxic effects in man cannot be verified by direct experiment and so extrapolation from the results of animal studies is essential. Of course the objective is to have as large a

margin of safety as possible. However when there is conflicting data does one use the single positive result or the **'weight' of all the data?** Inflated estimates of exposure may occur. **Epidemiology** may be useful for compounds that have been used for some time. Indeed, many compounds have never undergone a full range of toxicity tests (an estimated 70 per cent in the USA) and it would clearly be an enormous task to test all such compounds. Consequently, a reliance on epidemiology is unavoidable.

Conclusions

As yet, toxicologists only partially understand the mechanisms underlying relatively few toxic effects of chemicals. Consequently the assessment of risk to man will remain difficult and uncertain. The limitations need to be borne in mind by the public, by industrialists, economists and regulatory officials, but also by toxicologists themselves.

Perhaps the public expects too much from scientists in general and toxicologists in particular. Toxicology *cannot* provide all of the answers the public often demands as they are beyond current science. The public may demand **absolute safety** but this is an impossible dream. One of the duties of the toxicologist is to make sure the limitations are *understood*.

Perhaps the real crux of the problem of interpretation of toxicological data in the light of increasing and widespread exposure of humans to chemicals is the assessment of **risk versus benefit**. Although the public may not always be aware of the fact that chemicals confer benefits on society, and that there is a greater or lesser risk attached to their use, the benefits may be hard to quantify and compare with the risk. However, just as we take a quantifiable risk when we drive a car because its use is convenient and maybe essential, then we should apply similar principles to the chemicals we use. Unfortunately the risks and benefits may not always be equally shared, with one section of society reaping financial benefits while another risks the adverse effects.

Summary and learning objectives

Toxicity testing of chemicals is a *legal* requirement if humans or animals in the environment are likely to be exposed. This toxicity may be determined from epidemiology studies and clinical trials, *in vivo* studies in animals and studies *in vitro* but is mostly from animals.

Epidemiology (cohort, case control, cross sectional or ecological studies) may indicate relative or absolute risk. *In vivo* tests are carried out but questions must be asked (e.g. dosage size and frequency and physico-chemical properties, novelty) and biological considerations (e.g. species and sex of animal) addressed beforehand. The nature of the test will depend on the type of chemical, its use and the particular chemical. General tests used are *acute* (1 dose), *sub-chronic* (repeated, 28 or 90 days) and *chronic* (at least 12 months in rodents). More specific tests include those for *reproductive toxicity* (effects on male or female reproductive system), *teratogenicity* (effects on the embryo *in utero*) and *carcinogenicity* (ability to cause tumours) and *ecotoxicity* (e.g. effects on *Daphnia* and earthworms). For some chemicals (e.g. industrial chemicals) only acute tests may be needed for classification (e.g. non-toxic/very toxic). *Acute tests* will help define a dose–response relationship. *Sub-chronic* and *chronic studies* indicate target organ(s) toxicity, other pathological effects, blood level

and no observed effect level. Other specific *in vivo* studies will be carried out if necessary. Toxicity testing *in vivo* should consider the three Rs: *replacement*, *reduction* and *refinement*. Replacement means the use of *in vitro test* systems including those for mutagenicity involving bacteria (e.g. *Salmonella* in the *Ames* test), mammalian cells (mouse lymphoma, human lymphocytes) or insects (fruit flies). Testing for cytotoxicity may utilize mammalian-derived cells, mostly for screening out chemicals prior to *in vivo* evaluation or for evaluation of skin toxicity or allergenicity. There are significant limitations to *in vitro* tests (e.g. loss of enzyme activity). Reduction means using the minimum animals necessary and refinement means devising methods to gain the most information while causing the least distress.

Risks from chemical exposure must be assessed in relation to benefit.

Risk is the probability that an adverse effect will occur under specific exposure conditions.

Hazard is the capability of a substance to cause an adverse effect. *Risk assessment* is the process whereby exposure, hazard and risk are determined.

The *hazard* needs to be identified from human epidemiology, animal toxicity studies or *in vitro* studies. *Dose–response relationships* will also be determined from this information. For most chemicals a NOAEL or LOAEL can be determined. *Exposure assessment* and other aspects of risk assessment includes use of biomarkers of exposure, response and susceptibility and physico-chemical characteristics are important pieces of information.

Risk characterization involves integrating all the information and calculating parameters such as acceptable daily intake (ADI), tolerable daily intake (TDI) or threshold limit value (TLV) using the NOAEL and a safety or uncertainty factor. This is typically 100 (10 for species extrapolation, 10 for human variability). For carcinogens different models will be used to those exhibiting a threshold for effect (e.g. one-hit, multi-hit). Carcinogenicity testing requires lifetime studies *in vivo* in large numbers of animals often including the maximum tolerated dose.

Questions

Q1. Indicate which of the following are true or false:

  a acute toxicity studies are primarily for the determination of mutagenicity
  b sub-chronic toxicity tests are for the measurement of dose response
  c ecotoxicity studies may utilize tests in *Daphnia*
  d teratogenicity tests are part of reproductive toxicity studies.

Q2. Which of the following are important in risk assessment:

  a exposure level or dose
  b hazard
  c NOAEL
  d benefit
  e ADI
  f cost
  g TLV.

SHORT ANSWER QUESTIONS

Q3. Give four of the seven questions which should be asked before a toxicity study is carried out.

Q4. List the four types of epidemiological study.

Q5. Define the three Rs in relation to toxicity testing.

Q6. Define risk and hazard.

Bibliography

Alternatives in Animal Alternatives for Safety and Efficacy Testing, H. Salem and, S. A. Katz (Eds), revised edition (1997), Taylor & Francis. Covers the alternatives to animals for testing, minimizing numbers and discomfort, maximizing the information received.

AUER, C. M. and FIELDER, R. J. (1999) chapter 72, in *General and Applied Toxicology*, Ballantyne, B., Marrs, T. and Syversen, T. L. M. (Eds), 2nd edition, Basingstoke: Macmillan.

Biomarkers and Risk Assessment. Environmental Health Criteria 155, WHO, Geneva, 1993.

BROWN, V. K. (1988) *Acute and Sub-acute Toxicology*, London: Edward Arnold.

Chemical Risk Assessment, Training Module No. 3 UNEP/IPCS 1999, Geneva: WHO. An accessible source of information and teaching aid which can be obtained free from the IPCS, Geneva (ipcsmail@who.ch)

ECOBICHON, D. J. (1997) *The Basis of Toxicity Testing (Pharmacology and Toxicology)*, 2nd edition, CRC Press.

FAIRHURST, S. (1999) chapter 67, in *General and Applied Toxicology*, Ballantyne, B., Marrs, T. and Syversen, T. L. M. (Eds) 2nd edition, Basingstoke: Macmillan.

General and Applied Toxicology, Ballantyne, B., Marrs, T. and Syversen, T. L. M. (Eds), 2nd edition, 1999, Basingstoke: Macmillan. Various chapters in Part 8.

GRIFFIN, J. P. (1985) Predictive value of animal toxicity studies, *ATLA*, **12**, 163.

Hazardous chemicals in human and environmental health (2000) IPCS, Geneva: WHO. A simple but informative concise book, which can be obtained free from the IPCS, Geneva (ipcsmail@who.ch)

HEUVEL, M. J. Van Den, DAYAN, A. D. and SHILLAKER, R. O. (1987) Evaluation of the BTS approach to the testing of substances and preparations for their acute toxicity, *Human Toxicology*, **6**, 279.

HOMBURGER, F. (Ed.) (1983–) *Safety Evaluation and Regulation of Chemicals*, 3 vols, Basel: Karger.

LU, F. C. (1996) *Basic Toxicology*, 3rd edition, New York: Taylor & Francis.

MERRILL, R. A. (1996) Regulatory toxicology, in *Cassarett and Doull's Toxicology*, Klaassen, C. (Ed.), 5th edition, New York: Pergamon Press.

NIEHS (1987) Basic research in risk assessment, *Environmental Health Perspectives,* **76** (Dec).

Principles and Methods of Toxicology, A. W. Hayes (Ed.), 4th edition, 2001, Philadelphia: Taylor & Francis. Various chapters.

ROBERTS, C. N. (Ed.) (1989) *Risk Assessment – The Common Ground,* Eye, Suffolk: Life Science Research.

ROLOFF, M. V. (Ed.) (1987) *Human Risk Assessment. The Role of Animal Selection and Extrapolation,* Philadelphia: Taylor & Francis.

SCALA, R. A. (1991) Risk assessment, in *Cassarett and Doull's Toxicology,* Amdur, M. O., Doull, J. and Klaassen, C. (Eds), 4th edition, New York: Pergamon Press.

WALD, N. J. (1996) *The Epidemiological Approach*, 3rd edition, London: Wolfson Institute of Preventive Medicine.

WILKINSON, C. F. (1986) Risk assessment and regulatory policy, *Comments on Toxicology,* **1**, 1-21.

ZBINDON, G. and FLURY-REVERSI, M. (1981) Significance of the LD_{50} test for the toxicological evaluation of chemical substances, *Archives of Toxicology,* **47**, 77.

Answers to questions

Chapter 1

A1. (d) Potentiation.

The compound B is not toxic, yet when combined with A the toxicity is increased. Thus, compound B potentiates the toxicity of A. This is distinct from synergism where both compounds are toxic but the toxicity of the combination is more than the sum of the individual toxicities.

A2. (e) All of the above.

A properly designed and carefully executed and observed acute toxicity study may give information on all of these parameters. (The therapeutic index may be determined provided the ED_{50} is known.) The LD_{50} is now rarely required as an end in itself except for specific situations such as the design of pesticides. However, with a novel compound where the toxicity and lethality are unknown, doses that prove to be lethal may be administered to animals in preliminary toxicity studies. Consequently, an LD_{50} could be calculated from such data.

A3. (c) LD_{50}/ED_{50}.

Therefore the bigger the therapeutic index the safer the drug. A better and more discriminating definition would be TD_{50}/ED_{50} in which the toxicity rather than the lethality is used for the numerator.

SHORT ANSWER QUESTIONS

A4. (a) TD_{50} is the dose of a compound that is toxic to 50 per cent of the population exposed to that compound. The value is determined from the dosage–response relationship by interpolation (see Figure 1.5).

(b) Dosage (dose)–response relationship is the mathematical relationship between the dosage (dose) of a compound and the particular response measured. The response may be quantal (e.g. 'all-or-none' such as lethality) or graded (e.g. inhibition of an enzyme). The relationship is typically a sigmoid curve. This reflects the fact that there are doses that have no effect and those that have a maximal effect (see Figure 1.4).

(c) Therapeutic index is an index of relative toxicity for a drug. Calculated as the LD_{50} or TD_{50} divided by the ED_{50}. Thus the greater the number, the less toxic the drug is relative to the pharmacologically effective dose. This is reflected in Figure 1.5.

(d) NOEL (The No Observed Effect Level) is the dose or exposure level of a chemical which has no demonstrable effect on a biological system. (NOAEL: No Observed Adverse Effect Level.) The value may be derived from the dosage–response relationship. (See Figure 1.7.)

A5. Selective toxicity means that certain organisms are susceptible to a toxicant and others are not. For example, insects are susceptible to the toxicity of DDT and malathion whereas mammals are generally not. Bacteria are susceptible to drugs such as penicillin whilst humans are not. This selectivity in the toxic effects is therefore exploited in drugs used to fight infections, cancer and to remove pests such as insects. The basis of the selectivity may be metabolic or structural. For example the malathion is metabolized differently in insects to mammals and the bacterial cell wall is structurally different from the mammalian cell membrane and so is a target for penicillin.

A6. (a) The ED_{50} is the dose of a compound that causes an effect in 50 per cent of the organisms or a 50 per cent response. This is usually a pharmacological, as distinguished from a toxicological, effect. The ED_{50} may be determined in a population of organisms or in an *in vitro* system. It may be a quantal ('all-or-none') response such as presence or absence of a pharmacological change or a graded response observed in the effect (see Figure 1.5).

(b) The ADI is defined as the 'acceptable daily intake'. This is usually applied to food additives or contaminants (such as pesticides). It is the calculated amount of a substance to which humans can be permitted to be exposed safely. It is calculated from the No Observed Adverse Effect Level (NOAEL) thus:

$$ADI = \frac{NOAEL \text{ mg kg}^{-1} \text{day}^{-1}}{100}$$

The value of 100 is the safety factor that is applied. This takes into account the possible differences in susceptibility between the species used to determine the NOAEL and humans. A higher safety factor may be applied in some cases.

(c) The margin of safety is similar to the therapeutic index but more critical. Thus it is an indication of the difference between the dose or concentration of a drug required for the desired pharmacological effect and the dose associated with a toxic effect. It is calculated as follows:

$$\text{margin of safety} = \frac{TD_1}{ED_{99}} \text{ or } \frac{LD_1}{ED_{99}}$$

where TD_1 and LD_1 are the doses that are toxic or lethal for 1 per cent of the population exposed and the ED_{99} is the dose that is effective in 99 per cent of the population. (See Figure 1.5.)

The margin of safety is more critical than the therapeutic index because it takes into account possible overlap in the dose–response curves for pharmacological and toxicological effects.

Chapter 2

A1. (c) Potential to bioaccumulate.

The larger the partition coefficient the greater is the lipophilicity and this correlates with the bioaccumulation of the compound in fat tissue.

A2. (c) Weak organic acids

In the stomach the pH is around 2 and at this pH weak acids will be non-ionized. Therefore passive absorption of the non-ionized acid will occur in the stomach.

A3. (b) Sometimes larger than the total body volume.

When a drug is bound to tissue components or sequestered in a tissue such as adipose tissue, the plasma level may be very low. Therefore the calculation of volume of distribution ($V_D =$ dose/plasma level) yields a value which may be higher than the total body water. The volume of distribution may be equal to the total body water but this is not always the case.

A4. (f) The total body clearance. Although some of the other factors may have an effect on half-life, by definition the total body clearance is the major determining factor as this includes metabolism and excretion.

A5. (b) The drug is mostly metabolized by the gastrointestinal tract and/or liver before reaching the systemic circulation.

The 'first-pass effect' is where a drug is removed by metabolism in the organ(s)/tissues through which it passes during absorption and before reaching the systemic circulation. This is commonly the gastrointestinal tract and liver, but could also be the lungs or skin.

A6.   (b) False.

Non-ionized compounds are more readily absorbed by passive diffusion as they more readily pass through the lipid bilayer parts of biological membranes.

A7.   (b) False.

The binding of drugs to plasma proteins only rarely involves covalent binding. Usually ionic, hydrogen, hydrophobic or van der Waals' forces are involved.

A8.   C.

Both lipophilicity and resistance to metabolism will favour accumulation of chemicals in biological systems. The former will result in sequestration in adipose tissue, the latter will decrease removal of the chemical by metabolism to polar, hydrophilic metabolites and loss by excretion.

A9.   C.

Chemicals with a long half-life are more likely to accumulate on repeated dosing especially if the dosing interval is shorter than the half-life.

SHORT ANSWER QUESTIONS

A10.   (a) The volume of distribution (V_D) is the volume of body fluid in which a chemical is apparently distributed after administration to an animal. It is calculated from either the dose and plasma (blood) concentration at a single time point or from the dose, area under the curve (AUC) and elimination rate constant (k_{el}):

$$V_D = \frac{\text{dose (mg)}}{\text{plasma concentration (mg L}^{-1})}$$

The units are therefore in litres.

The volume of distribution does not necessarily equal a compartment and so may have a value higher than the total body water (40 litres for a human). This occurs if the plasma level is low, as when a drug is sequestered such as in adipose tissue. V_D is therefore known as apparent volume of distribution. The volume of distribution should not be calculated after the drug is administered orally as there may be incomplete absorption and/or first-pass metabolism.

(b) Drugs normally bind to plasma proteins non-covalently and in one of four ways:

(i)   by ionic bonds in which there is bonding between charged groups or atoms and opposite charges on the protein.

(ii) by hydrogen bonds where a hydrogen atom attached to an electronegative atom (e.g. oxygen) is shared with another electronegative atom.

(iii) by hydrophobic interactions in which two non-polar, hydrophilic groups associate and mutually repel water.

(iv) by van der Waals' forces: these are weak forces acting between the nucleus of one atom and the electrons of another.

There may be several molecules of drug bound to one protein molecule and strength may vary depending on the type of binding. However, binding is normally reversible. The protein commonly involved in binding is albumin. Binding to plasma proteins may increase the half-life and limit the distribution and metabolism of a drug. Drugs bound to plasma proteins may be displaced by other drugs, leading to a large rise in the free concentration in the plasma. Similarly increasing the dose of a drug which is bound extensively to plasma proteins may saturate the binding sites and lead to a sudden increase in plasma level.

(c) The first-pass effect is the extensive metabolism of a drug either by the organ of absorption or the liver following oral administration. This may lead to the situation where very little of the parent drug is distributed around the body. Thus after oral absorption a drug may be metabolized by the gastrointestinal tract and/or the liver before reaching the systemic circulation. Therefore if the parent drug is active, little may reach the target site. If the metabolism is saturable, however, increasing the dose may dramatically increase the systemic exposure. The lungs and skin, the other organs of absorption, may also carry out first-pass metabolism. Figure 2.10 shows the effect of the first-pass metabolism of a compound after oral and intravenous administration.

(d) Fick's law of diffusion describes the relationship between the rate of diffusion of a chemical across a membrane and certain characteristics of the membrane. In the context of toxicology and drug disposition it relates to passage across a cell membrane by simple diffusion. Thus:

$$\text{rate of diffusion } = KA(C_2 - C_1)$$

where K is the diffusion coefficient, A is the surface area, C_2 is the concentration of compound outside the membrane, C_1 is the concentration of compound on the inside of the membrane. The diffusion coefficient will incorporate physico-chemical characteristics of the chemical such as lipophilicity, size, shape, etc.

A11. (a) The pH partition theory states that only non-ionized lipid soluble compounds will be absorbed by passive diffusion down a concentration gradient. For absorption of a compound to occur through a biological membrane the compound must be lipid soluble and the concentration on the inside of the membrane should be lower than on the outside. Compounds that are ionized at the pH of the biological environment will not normally be able to pass through the membrane by passive diffusion although they may be substrates for active transport processes.

(b) Plasma half-life ($t_{\frac{1}{2}}$) is the time taken for the concentration of a drug in the plasma (blood) to decrease by half from a given point. It reflects the rates at which the various *in vivo* dynamic processes of distribution, metabolism and excretion are taking place. It

can be determined from a plot of the plasma level against time by measurement (see Figure 2.10) or from the equation:

$$\text{half-life} = \frac{0.693}{k_{el}}$$

where k_{el} is determined from the slope of the graph log plasma concentration vs time (slope $= -k_{el}/2.303$).

The half-life is an important measurement as changes in this parameter may reflect, for example, saturation of metabolism or excretion. A knowledge of the half-life is also important in relation to repeat dosing with a drug. If the dosing interval is shorter than the half-life then accumulation will occur. (See Figure 2.11.)

(c) Plasma clearance is a derived parameter and is an indication of the rate of removal of a drug from the blood or other body fluid by excretion or metabolism. It is calculated from the area under the plasma concentration vs time curve (AUC):

$$\text{clearance} = \frac{\text{dose}}{\text{AUC}}$$

Therefore, the units are volume/unit time, e.g. ml min^{-1}. Thus a plasma clearance of 100 ml min^{-1} means that 100 ml of plasma is completely cleared of the drug every minute. Therefore the higher the clearance, the more efficiently and rapidly a chemical is removed from the fluid.

(d) The term enterohepatic recirculation describes the process whereby a chemical in the body is secreted from the liver into the bile, passes into the small intestine and is then reabsorbed into the blood stream. For example, the chemical may be secreted into bile as a polar conjugate following metabolism in the liver. Then when the bile enters the intestine this conjugate is cleaved by bacterial metabolism and the original drug or other fragment is reabsorbed from the intestine and re-enters the liver via the portal circulation. (See Figure 2.13.) This process may be repeated several times and therefore it prolongs the exposure of the liver and rest of the body to the compound. If the compound has been administered orally, very little may reach the systemic circulation. The plasma level profile may reflect the process by showing peaks at various times, corresponding to reabsorption, rather than a smooth decline.

Chapter 3

A1. (d) Altered chemical structure.

Metabolism by definition involves alteration of the chemical structure of a drug. Although increased excretion and decreased toxicity may often also occur this does not always happen and increased toxicity may result.

A2. (c) Is a central part of the drug metabolizing system.

Cytochrome P450 is the most important enzyme involved in drug metabolism. It is localized in the smooth endoplasmic reticulum and catalyses most of the phase 1 oxidation reactions.

A3. (d) The addition of an endogenous moiety.

Phase 2 metabolic transformations involve addition of a moiety derived endogenously which usually increases the polarity and water solubility. The moieties commonly involved are glucuronic acid, sulphate, glutathione and amino acids such as glycine.

A4. (b) A tripeptide.

Glutathione is composed of three amino acids: glutamic acid, cysteine and glycine (glutamyl-cysteinyl-glycine) abbreviated glu-cys-gly. It is involved in detoxication by conjugating with reactive metabolites, by reducing reactive metabolites and by reacting with and donating a hydrogen atom to free radicals.

A5. (a) True.

Cytochrome P450 catalyses phase 1 oxidation reactions.

A6. E.

All of these are involved in the operation of the microsomal enzyme system.

A7. (d) An inherited trait affecting a particular metabolic reaction.

The acetylation reaction in which the acetyl group (CH_3CO) is added to an amine, hydrazine or sulphonamide group is subject to genetic variation in humans. There are two phenotypes, rapid and slow acetylators which is a single gene trait governed by simple Mendelian inheritance with the rapid acetylator trait being dominant. This genetic trait results in a difference in the enzyme between the two phenotypes such that in the slow acetylators the enzyme, *N*-acetyltransferase (NAT2), catalyses the acetylation of substrates less efficiently than in the rapid acetylators. In the slow acetylators there are mutations in the gene coding for the enzyme, resulting in a relatively dysfunctional enzyme.

A8. (a) An increase in the synthesis of the enzyme.

Although the activity (and substrate specificity) of the enzyme may seem to be altered, in fact it is the synthesis of particular isozymes and their proportions which are altered. With some inducers liver weight and bile flow are increased, but not all inducers cause this.

SHORT ANSWER QUESTIONS

A9. (a) Dealkylation is the removal of an alkyl (usually a methyl or ethyl group) from a molecule. The alkyl group may be attached to a nitrogen, sulphur or oxygen atom as indicated below. The dealkylation reaction is catalyzed by the microsomal mono-oxygenase enzyme cytochrome P450 and involves an initial oxidation of the alkyl carbon atom followed by a rearrangement with loss of the oxidized alkyl group as an aldehyde (e.g. methanal or ethanal as indicated below). The other product is either an alcohol, thiol or amine as shown below:

$$R - O - C_2H_5 \rightarrow R - OH + CH_3CHO$$
$$R - NH - CH_3 \rightarrow R - NH_2 + HCHO$$
$$R - S - CH_3 \rightarrow R - SH + HCHO$$

(b) Alcohol dehydrogenase is an enzyme found in many animal species that catalyzes the oxidation of alcohols to aldehydes. The coenzyme NADH is also required. There are several isoenzymes and a wide variety of alcohols are substrates. The enzyme is found particularly in the liver. There is evidence to suggest that there may be ethnic variations in the enzyme activity with Canadian Indians having reduced ability to metabolize ethanol.

(c) Glucuronic acid conjugation is the combination of certain foreign compounds with glucuronic acid to form glucuronides. Normally a carboxylic acid group or a hydroxyl group is conjugated to form ester or ether glucuronides. Occasionally thiol and NH glucuronides may be formed. The conjugates are water soluble and therefore readily excreted. The conjugation is catalyzed by one of a group of glucuronosyltransferases. Glucuronic acid is a six carbon carbohydrate molecule formed from glucose-1-phosphate. For conjugation it is combined with uridine diphosphate (UDP) as UDP-glucuronic acid. (See Figure 3.15.)

(d) Phase 1 metabolism refers to the first stage in the biotransformation of a foreign compound. The product will normally have a functional group added or an existing one modified that can be used as a 'handle' for a second endogenous group, derived from intermediary metabolism, such as glucuronic acid to be added in phase 2 metabolism. (See Figure 3.3.)

A10. (a) The ethnic background of a human individual may be an important determinant of their response to drugs and other chemicals. This may be due to a difference in sensitivity/ susceptibility or to a difference in disposition. Glucose-6-phosphate dehydrogenase deficiency increases susceptibility to certain drugs such as primaquine, resulting in haemolytic anaemia. This deficiency is found in male individuals of a particular ethnic origin, such as those who inhabit or derive from the eastern Mediterranean such as Sephardic Jews from Kurdistan. Altered disposition in particular ethnic groups often occurs as a result of differences in enzymes. For example, the acetylator phenotype is differently distributed in Orientals compared with Egyptians, being mostly fast acetylators in the former but slow acetylators in the latter.

(b) The cytochrome P450 system, responsible for metabolizing many drugs, consists of many isozymes. These have different substrate specificities and there is variation in the activity of these isozymes between species and individuals. Therefore absence of a particular isozyme in an individual or species might make them more susceptible to drug toxicity if the particular isozyme was responsible for a detoxication pathway. Conversely, the individual or species might be less susceptible to a particular drug toxicity. The same also applies to susceptibility of a tissue to a particular drug toxicity, as isozymes vary in proportions between tissues within the same animal.

(c) The phenomenon of enzyme induction is the apparent increase in activity of an enzyme following the exposure of the animal to a xenobiotic. For example, repeated exposure to phenobarbital leads to an apparent increase in the activity of certain cytochrome P450 isozymes. This can be shown to occur with other enzymes involved with drug metabolism such as glucuronosyltransferase. The result is that the metabolism and therefore toxicity of a drug may be increased or decreased. This will depend on whether the drug or a metabolite is responsible for the toxic effect. For example, paracetamol toxicity to the liver is increased by induction of cytochrome P450 with phenobarbital in some species.

(d) Acetylator phenotype is a genetically determined characteristic in humans that determines the extent of acetylation of certain drugs. Isoniazid acetylation is affected by this phenotype. The phenotype is the result of a genetic difference between individuals resulting from mutations in the gene coding for *N*-acetyltransferase 2. Thus slow acetylators have less functional enzyme than fast acetylators. The result is that detoxication by acetylation of hydrazines, sulphonamides and amines is decreased in slow acetylators. Toxic effects such as hydralazine-induced lupus and isoniazid-induced peripheral neuropathy are more common in the slow phenotype.

Chapter 4

A1. (b) Dose.

Although all of the other factors may affect toxicity, the most important is the dose as toxicity is a relative phenomenon. Therefore at low enough doses there will be no toxic effect.

A2. (b) The liver metabolizes chemicals and this activity often makes it a target for toxicity. This may be due to the production of reactive metabolites or because its other metabolic activities are affected.

(c) The blood that is supplied to the liver is partly derived from the gut via the portal vein. Therefore chemicals absorbed from the gut will be presented to the liver. If toxic they may damage the liver tissue.

(d) The liver produces bile into which chemicals are excreted. Consequently, high concentrations of certain chemicals may occur in the bile and damage the bile duct. Alternatively, chemicals that are excreted into the bile via active transport, may, under conditions of high dosage, saturate

the transport processes and accumulate in the liver, thereby causing damage.

A3. (e) Steatosis. Fatty liver or steatosis is the most common response of the liver to exposure to chemicals. This is because the liver is the primary site of fat metabolism in the mammalian body and this is easily disrupted by chemicals in various ways.

A4. (b) Immunosuppression. This is where the function of the immune system is reduced by a chemical such as dioxin or benzene which damages the thymus and bone marrow, respectively.

(d) Autoimmune reactions. These are immune-mediated reactions where the immune system attacks the structure of the body itself. An example is halothane-induced hepatic damage.

A5. (a) Death.

Although teratogens may cause all of these effects, especially growth retardation during the first stage of pregnancy before implantation, organogenesis or functional maturation, the fertilized egg is more likely to suffer death following exposure to a chemical.

A6.

Aneuploidization	loss or acquisition of a complete chromosome
Clastogenesis	loss, addition or rearrangement of parts of chromosomes
Mutagenesis	addition to or alteration of the number of base pairs

A7. (a) To indicate exposure has occurred. (d) To measure response and susceptibility. Biomarkers are biochemical indicators of the exposure, the response or the susceptibility to chemicals.

SHORT ANSWER QUESTIONS

A8. Direct toxic action: tissue lesions e.g. paracetamol-induced liver damage; biochemical lesions, e.g. fluoroacetate interference with the TCA cycle leading to death from cardiac arrest; pharmacological/physiological effects, e.g. malathion causing exaggerated effects of acetylcholine; immunotoxicity, e.g. allergic responses caused by exposure to penicillin; teratogenicity, e.g. thalidomide-induced birth defects; genetic toxicity, e.g. 5-bromouracil becomes incorporated into replicating DNA and this leads to mutations (base-pair transformations); carcinogenicity, e.g. vinyl chloride and aflatoxin both cause liver cancer.

A9. Immunosuppression, autoimmune responses, hypersensitivity and allergic reactions. Immunosuppression is where the function of the immune system is reduced by a chemical such as dioxin or benzene which damage the thymus and bone marrow, respectively. Autoimmunity is where the immune system damages or destroys the structure of the body itself such as occurs in halothane hepatoxicity. Hypersensitivity is where the immune system recognizes that a chemical is foreign and mounts a response involving antibodies in a humoral response or lymphocytes in a cell-mediated response. Hydralazine-induced lupus is a response in which antibodies and an antibody–antigen complex is formed. An allergic reaction is where the immune system recognizes that a substance is foreign and an immune reaction is mounted, for example as occurs with foreign proteins such as pollen or those devised to be used as drugs.

A10. The first stage is initiation, in which the chemical or a reactive metabolite interacts with DNA. The second stage is promotion in which the initiated cell undergoes division and a clone of initiated/altered cells is produced. Finally, the third stage is where the clone of cells undergoes progressions in which the neoplastic cells may become a malignant tumour, growth increases and the cells become malignant and invade tissue.

Chapter 5

A1. E.

After overdoses or inappropriate doses of a drug the pharmacological effect may be exaggerated, for example excessive lowering of blood pressure. This is an adverse effect. Sometimes a drug may cause an adverse effect after therapeutic doses in particularly susceptible individuals. This is an idiosyncrasy. Inappropriate doses of a drug may cause unwanted effects not related to the expected/desired pharmacological effect of that drug. Occasionally there may be an interaction between a drug and a dietary constituent such as between monoamine oxidase inhibitor drugs and amines in foodstuffs such as cheese.

A2. (d) Metabolic activation by the microsomal enzymes.

Although (a) and (c) are also true, metabolic activation to a reactive benzoquinoneimine, which interacts with tissue components, is the cause of the toxicity. (See Figure 5.1.)

A3. (a), (b), (c). There are a number of predisposing factors in hydralazine toxicity. These include the acetylator phenotype, gender and dose. The toxicity or adverse effect is almost exclusively confined to the slow acetylator. The toxicity is more common in females than males. The adverse effect is more likely to occur at higher doses (although the severity of the effect does not seem to be related to the dose).

A4. (c) Thalidomide was a sedative drug used for the relief of morning sickness in pregnant women. It caused malformations in babies born to mothers who took the drug during the susceptible period (3rd to 8th week of pregnancy). The malformations were shortened arms and legs, known as phocomelia. The S isomer of the drug is more active than the R isomer. Pregnant rats were not susceptible to this effect.

A5. (c) Halothane, an anaesthetic drug may occasionally cause severe liver damage in patients. This is more common in females than males. The mechanism involves metabolism by cytochrome P450 and production of an antigenic conjugate. The immune response involves T-lymphocytes as well as antibodies. It is an auto-immune reaction. (See Figure 5.5.)

SHORT ANSWER QUESTION

A6. Aspirin is mainly metabolized to salicylate. The distribution of salicylate into tissues and its excretion into urine are sensitive to pH. This is because only the ionized form of salicylate enters tissues and especially the brain. However, the brain in particular is sensitive to the toxic effects of salicylate. When plasma pH drops, as a result of salicylate poisoning, this distribution into the brain increases. Similarly, excretion into urine is reduced if urinary pH becomes more acidic. Raising the pH of plasma and urine with bicarbonate is therefore the central part of treatment of aspirin poisoning. (See Figure 5.3.)

Chapter 6

A1. (c) Dermatitis is a common reaction to the metal nickel.

A2. (a), (b), (c) and (d) are all known carcinogens. Cadmium is not known to be a carcinogen in man but asbestos, 2-naphthylamine and vinyl chloride are associated with lung cancer (mesothelioma), bladder cancer and liver cancer (haemangiosarcoma) in man, respectively.

A3. (c) The NOAEL or No Observed Adverse Effect Level is needed to determine the Threshold Limit Value (TLV) for an industrial chemical. This is unusually divided by a safety factor to give the TLV. The latency period for the effect and half-life would be included in the NOAEL. The daily exposure level may be the same as, less or more than the TLV depending on the particular circumstances.

A4. The toxicity of asbestos is affected by (a), (b), (c), (d) and (e).

A5. (c) Both vinyl chloride and cadmium affect bones, albeit in different ways.

SHORT ANSWER QUESTION

A6. 2-Naphthylamine undergoes hydroxylation on the nitrogen atom catalyzed by cytochrome P450 and the N-hydroxy product is conjugated with glucuronic acid. This conjugate is excreted into the urine but is relatively unstable and under the acidic conditions of the urine is hydrolyzed to yield a reactive metabolite. This reacts with DNA in the cells of the bladder that are exposed leading to the formation of cancer. However, 2-naphthylamine is also acetylated on the nitrogen atom and this is a detoxication reaction as hydroylation and reactive metabolite formation do not subsequently occur. Therefore the fast acetylator phenotype individual is less at risk than the slow acetylator.

Chapter 7

A1.

Erythrosine	colouring agent
Monosodium glutamate	flavour enhancer
Cinnamaldehyde	flavour
Butylated hydroxytoluene	anti-oxidant
Benzoyl peroxide	bleach

A2. Tartrazine is a colouring agent which may cause urticaria (b) and is reduced by gut bacteria (c). It is also known as E102. Tartrazine sensitivity is often related to aspirin tolerance.

A3. (a), (d) and (e) are true. Saccharin may cause bladder tumours in rats at very high doses. Saturation kinetics occurs at high doses, which may account for the bladder tumours at these doses. It has low toxicity and although it was banned from use under the Delaney Clause for a while it is now allowed for use.

A4. (d) Is true, (a),(b) and (c) are false. Adulterated rape-seed oil was sold for use as cooking oil. The rape-seed oil was for industrial use and had been adulterated with the addition of aniline. There were a number of symptoms including pulmonary oedema and muscular atrophy.

SHORT ANSWER QUESTION

A5. Aflatoxin. These are toxins produced by a mould (*Aspergillus flavus*) that grows on foodstuffs such as peanuts when stored in damp, warm conditions. Aflatoxin B_1 is a potent liver carcinogen. The mechanism involves metabolism to a chemically reactive intermediate, an epoxide, which interacts with DNA.

Ptaquiloside. This is a toxin which occurs in naturally in edible bracken fern shoots. It causes throat cancer in humans. In animals it causes intestinal and bladder cancer. A breakdown product of ptaquiloside is responsible, reacting with adenine in DNA and causing DNA strand breakage.

Botulinum toxin. This is one of the most potent toxins known. It is produced by the anaerobic bacterium *Clostridium botulinum*. It may contaminate tinned and bottled food, although it is destroyed by heating. It acts by binding irreversibly to the nerve terminals, preventing the release of acetylcholine. This causes paralysis and fatal cessation of breathing.

Chapter 8

A1. (b) and (d) are true; (a), (c), (e), (f) and (g) are false.

DDT is an organochlorine pesticide, which has low mammalian toxicity and does not destroy plants. Unlike organophosphates it does not inhibit cholinesterases. It is not directly toxic to eggs although it may contribute to their breakage as a result of eggshell thinning.

A2. Parathion is an organophosphate insecticide which is toxic to humans. Parathion is metabolized to paraoxon which inhibits cholinesterases leading to elevated levels of acetylcholine which causes excessive cholinergic stimulation and symptoms such as bronchoconstriction. (See Figure 8.4.)

True: (d) and (e). False: (a)–(c).

A3. Paraquat

True: (c) and (d). False: (a), (b), (e) and (f).

Paraquat is a bipyridyl herbicide. It is actively taken up into lung tissue by the putrescine uptake system. It is concentrated in the lungs where it causes lipid peroxidation, the production of active oxygen species and fibrosis. The active oxygen species are detoxified by superoxide dismutase (SOD) but this is overwhelmed when large amounts of paraquat are ingested. (See Figure 8.6.)

SHORT ANSWER QUESTION

A4. Fluoroacetate is toxic because it is incorporated into intermediary metabolism, being first converted to fluoroacetyl CoA. This is incorporated into the tricarboxylic acid cycle, forming fluorocitrate. This analogue of citrate, however, cannot be further metabolized by the next step to cis-aconitate as the fluorine atom cannot be removed. Therefore the tricarboxylic acid cycle is blocked, ATP production compromised and mammals die of heart failure.

Chapter 9

A.1 True: (b), (c), (e). False: (a), (d).

Inorganic lead is present in cigarette smoke and can be absorbed as particles of lead oxide for example through the lungs. It interferes with the synthesis of haem, some of which occurs in the mitochondria. The result is a reduction of haemoglobin which leads to damage to red cells. Organic lead such as that added to petrol, is toxic to the central nervous system.

A2. (a), (b), (c) are not true; (d) and (e) are true.

Mercury binds to SH groups and organic mercury has a long half-life. Metallic mercury easily vaporizes and the vapour can be readily absorbed where it is toxic to a variety of tissues including the central nervous system. Inorganic mercury is especially toxic to the kidney.

A3. (f) is true; (a), (b), (c), (d) and (e) are false.

The great smog in London was in 1952. Photochemical smog contains ozone, nitrogen oxides and hydrocarbons. Ozone is an irritant,

toxic gas. PM10 is the name of very small particles (diameter less than 10 μm) that are believed to be responsible for lung disease. Acid rain results from the production of sulphur dioxide and nitrogen oxides. It is caused by the wet precipitation of sulphuric and nitric acids and the dry precipitation of sulphur dioxide and nitrogen oxides.

Reducing smog is largely the result of burning of fossil fuels and has high levels of sulphur dioxide and particulates.

A4. True: (c) and (e). False: (a), (b) and (d).

DDT is an insecticide, not especially toxic to birds or chicks directly. However, its metabolite DDE is responsible for causing eggshell thinning. This results in egg breakage and loss of chicks. By killing insects of many types, DDT also reduces the food supply of some birds.

SHORT ANSWER QUESTION

A5. Bioaccumulation is the accumulation of a chemical substance in a biological organism. This is usually a reflection of the lipophilicity of the compound.

Biomagnification is the process whereby the concentration of a chemical substance in the organisms in a food chain increases towards the top of the chain. Thus, the predator at the top of the food chain will have the highest concentration of pollutant.

For a compound to bioaccumulate it should be lipid soluble rather than water soluble. For example, the pesticide DDT will bioaccumulate in organisms exposed to it as it dissolves in the fat in adipose tissue. Second, the compound should be resistant to metabolism and therefore poorly excreted so that it is eliminated slowly from the organism. For example, polybrominated biphenyl compounds, such as those that contaminated livestock and people in Michigan in 1973, are very resistant to metabolism, are eliminated extremely slowly and so have very long half-lives. Continued exposure to such compounds will therefore result in accumulation in fat tissue.

Chapter 10

A1. True: (c) and (e). False: (a), (b) and (d).

Pyrrolizidine alkaloids are found in plants such as *Heliotropium* species. These compounds cause liver and lung damage. *Amanita phalloides* is a toxin found in the Death Cap mushroom. It causes liver damage which may be fatal. Botulinum toxin is produced by the anaerobic bacterium *Clostridium botulinum* and is highly toxic, causing paralysis. Ricin is the most toxic substance known and is found naturally in the castor bean. Fluoroacetate occurs naturally in certain plants in South Africa and Australia.

A2. True: (b) and (d). False (a) and (c).

Tetrodotoxin is a toxin found in the Puffer fish and Californian newt. It is highly potent, causing muscle paralysis. The toxin selectively blocks sodium channels along the axon, blocking transmission of the action potential.

SHORT ANSWER QUESTION

A3. Botulinum toxin causes irreversible blockade of the motor nerve terminal at the myoneural junction. This prevents the release of acetylcholine and the muscle behaves as if denervated. The victim therefore suffers paralysis and may have difficulty in breathing which can be fatal if severe.

Chapter 11

A1. True: (b). False: (a), (c), (d) and (e).

Ethylene glycol toxicity requires metabolism by the enzyme alcohol dehydrogenase. Ethanol is also metabolized by this enzyme and so when administered to a poisoned patient ethanol competes for the enzyme and blocks the metabolism of the ethylene glycol.

A2. True: (b), (d). False: (a), (c), and (e).

Carbon monoxide binds to haemoglobin more strongly than oxygen and forms carboxyhaemoglobin. The lack of oxygen in the tissues results in damage, especially to those that have a high demand for oxygen such as the brain and heart. Death is usually due to respiratory failure. Carbon monoxide will also bind to other haem proteins such as cytochromes. The lack of oxygen leads to anaerobic respiration and hence lactic acidosis.

A3. True: (a), (b). False: (c), (d) and (e).

Ethylene glycol is a dihydric alcohol which is metabolized by alcohol dehydrogenase to an aldehyde and then (via aldehyde dehydrogenase) subsequently to an acid. The final product is oxalic acid. This may crystallize in the brain. The increased production of NADH as a result of metabolism leads to excessive production of lactic acid and the presence of acidic metabolites causes acidosis.

A4. True: (a) and (f). False: (b), (c), (d), (e).

Some solvents may sensitize the myocardium leading to sudden death from heart attack in apparently healthy young people who have engaged in solvent abuse.
Alcohol depresses the central nervous system, especially at high doses. Alcohol is metabolized to acetic acid. The major target for methanol is the eye – it causes blindness. Large doses of alcohol lower blood sugar (hypoglycaemia).

A5. (b), (d) and (e). Dicobalt edetate, a chelating agent, is used as an antidote to cyanide poisoning. N-acetylcysteine is used as an antidote for paracetamol overdose as it helps to restore the glutathione that is depleted by paracetamol. Pralidoxime is used as an antidote to organophosphate poisoning, as it binds the organophosphate in preference to the acetylcholinesterase enzyme.

SHORT ANSWER QUESTION

A6. General treatments for poisoning include the use of emetics to cause vomiting and so rid the stomach of the poison; gastric lavage to wash the poison out of the stomach; absorbants which are given orally to the patient and absorb the poison in the stomach. Enhancing excretion may be used which involves administration of aqueous solutions by mouth or intravenously (forced diuresis) to increase urine flow. If bicarbonate or ammonium chloride are included in the aqueous fluid then the pH of the urine is made more basic or acidic, respectively. This change will facilitate the excretion of acids or bases, respectively.

Extraction of the poison from the blood may be used in severe cases and involves either haemoperfusion or haemodialysis.

Chapter 12

A1. True: (c) and (d). False: (a) and (b).

Acute toxicity studies are to define the toxicity and determine a dose–response relationship. Sub-chronic studies are for the determination of short-term repeated exposure. Ecotoxicity studies use the small water organism *Daphnia* as a test species. Teratogenicity studies are for the determination of the effect of a compound on the developing organism *in utero.*

A2. True: (a), (b), (c) and (d). False: (e), (f) and (g)

SHORT ANSWER QUESTIONS

A3. The following are the seven questions:

1 Is it a novel compound or has it been used before?
2 Is it to be released into the environment?
3 Is it to be added to human food?
4 Is it to be given as a single dose or repeatedly?
5 At what dosage level is it to be administered?
6 What age group will be exposed?
7 Are women of childbearing age likely to be exposed?

A4. The four types of epidemiological studies are: cohort studies, case-control studies, cross-sectional studies, ecological studies.

A5. The three Rs relate to the use of animals in toxicity testing. They are *replacement* of animals with alternatives such as *in vitro* systems; *reduction* of numbers of animals used by careful design of experiments and *refinement* of the techniques used to ensure greater animal welfare.

A6. *Risk* is defined as the probability that a hazard will cause an adverse effect under specific exposure conditions.

Risk may also be defined in the following way:

Risk = hazard × exposure.

Hazard is defined as the capability of a substance to cause an adverse effect. Conversely safety may be defined as 'the practical certainty that adverse effects will not occur when the substance is used in the manner and quantity proposed for its use'.

Glossary

Acidosis/alkalosis The condition when the pH of the blood falls/rises outside the normal acceptable limits.

Acid rain The deposition of acids (sulphuric and nitric) in rain and also the dry deposition of sulphur dioxide and nitrogen oxides.

Acute Short-term exposure or response.

Additive When the toxic effect of a mixture is equal to the sum of the toxicities of the components.

ADI The Acceptable Daily Intake. 'The daily intake of a chemical which during an entire lifetime appears to be without appreciable risk on the basis of all the known facts at the time.'

Aerobic/ anaerobic A process carried out in the presence/absence of air.

Aerosol A colloidal system with a gas as the dispersion medium (such as a fog or mist of droplets or particles).

Ah receptor A protein which binds polycyclic hydrocarbons such as dioxin (TCDD). Binding to this receptor is part of the process of induction of xenobiotic metabolizing enzymes.

Allergic reaction A reaction to a foreign agent giving rise to a hypersensitive state, mediated via an immunological mechanism and resulting in a particular series of responses.

Anaphylactic reaction A type I immunological response.

Aneuploidy Increase or decrease in the number of chromosomes of an organism.

Anoxia Absence of oxygen in the tissues.

Antagonism When the toxic effect of a mixture is less than the sum of the toxicities of the components.

Antibody A protein produced by lymphoid tissue in response to, and specific for, a foreign substance or antigen.

Anticoagulant A substance which inhibits the normal process of blood clotting.

Antidote A substance which specifically blocks or reduces the action of a poison.

Antigen A protein or other macromolecule which is recognized as foreign by the immune system in an animal.

Antiport Membrane carrier system in which two substances are transported in opposite directions.

Apoptosis Programmed cell death.

Asbestosis Damage to the lungs caused specifically by exposure to, and inhalation of, asbestos fibres.

Ataxia Failure of muscular coordination.

AUC Area under the curve when the plasma (blood) concentration of a substance is plotted against time.

β-adrenoceptors An autonomic receptor of which there are two types, β_1 and β_2.

Bioaccumulation The accumulation of a substance in a biological organism, usually due to its lipophilicity (q.v.).

Biomagnification The process whereby the concentration of a pollutant in organisms in a food chain increases towards the top of that chain. Thus the predator at the top of the food chain will have the highest concentration of pollutant.

Biomarker A biochemical or biological marker of exposure, response or susceptibility to chemicals.

Blebbing The appearance of blebs (protrusions) on the surface of cells in response to stress (e.g. chemicals).

Blood–brain barrier A description of the inability of many substances to pass from the blood to the tissues of the brain.

BOD Biochemical Oxygen Demand. This measurement indicates the ability of micro-organisms to metabolize an organic substance in the presence of oxygen and therefore the potential for depletion of oxygen by the substance.

Bronchocarcinoma Cancer of the lung.

Bronchoconstriction Constriction of the airways in the lungs due to exposure to irritant chemicals or to an immunological reaction involving release of inflammatory mediators.

Carcinogen/carcinogenic A substance/property of a substance which causes cancer when administered to an organism.

Cardiac arrythmias Abnormal beating rhythms in the heart.

Cardiac output The volume of blood pumped by the heart in one cycle.

Cerebral palsy A motor disorder due to damage to the brain.

Cholinergic stimulation Stimulation of the nerve fibres utilizing acetylcholine as a neurotransmitter.

Chronic (lifetime) Long-term exposure or response.

Cirrhosis Liver disease characterized by loss of the normal microscopic lobular structure with fibrosis and nodular regeneration. Usually the result of chronic injury to tissue.

Clastogenesis Occurrence of chromosomal breaks which result in a gain, loss or rearrangement of pieces of chromosomes.

Clearance The volume of plasma cleared of a substance in unit time.

Clinical trials The initial studies carried out with a drug in human subjects.

COD Chemical Oxygen Demand. The amount of oxygen required to oxidize the substance chemically.

COD/BOD The ratio of COD to BOD gives an indication of the biodegradability of the substance.

Collagen A fibrous protein.

Complement A series of proteins found in extracellular fluids and involved in certain immunological reactions.

Cyanosis The pathological condition where there is an excessive concentration of reduced haemoglobin in the blood.

Cytochrome a_3 A haem-containing enzyme which is part of the cytochrome c oxidase complex, the terminal cytochrome in the mitochondrial electron transport chain.

Cytological examination Examination of cells or examination for the presence of cells in urine.

Cytosol The internal part of the cell excluding the organelles.

Delaney Amendment Amendment to the Food, Drug and Cosmetic Act of the Food and Drug Administration of the United States. The amendment states that food additives which cause cancer in humans or animals at any level shall not be considered safe and are, therefore, prohibited.

Dermatitis Inflammation of the skin.

Detritivore food chain An animal which uses decaying organic matter as a food source, after the initial breakdown of the material by decomposers such as bacteria and fungi is known as a 'detritivore.' The type of food chain which relies on decaying organic matter for its primary energy source is known as a 'detritivore food chain.'

Dinoflagellates Single-celled marine algae possessing two flagella.

Disulphide bridge A sulphur-sulphur bond (S-S) such as occurs commonly in proteins.

Dominant lethal assay A test designed to detect the effects of substances on the germ cells of male animals which are exposed and then mated with untreated females. The number of dead implantations or preimplantation losses in the pregnant females are then determined. The effects are usually due to chromosome damage.

ED_{50} The dose which is pharmacologically effective for 50 per cent of the population exposed to the substance *or* a 50 per cent response in a biological system which is exposed to the substance.

Electrophilic A chemical description of a substance which seeks out a group or molecular position which has a preponderance of electrons and so is negatively charged.

Encephalopathy A degenerative disease of the brain.

Endocrine disruptor An exogenous substance which causes changes in endocrine function leading to adverse effects in an animal or its offspring.

Endogenous Part of the internal environment of a living organism.

Enterohepatic recirculation The cycling of a substance from the blood into the liver, then into the bile and gastrointestinal tract. This is followed by re-uptake into the bloodstream from the gastrointestinal tract possibly after chemical or enzymatic breakdown.

Epidemiology The study of diseases in populations.

Epigenetic When used as a description of a carcinogen or of mechanisms of carcinogenesis this means that interaction with genetic material, such as to yield a mutation, is not involved.

ER Endoplasmic reticulum. This may be divided into rough ER with attendant ribosomes involved with protein synthesis and smooth ER where cytochrome P450 and many other drug metabolizing enzymes are located.

Eutrophication Increased nutrient concentration in water resulting in the overgrowth of plants such as algae giving rise to a depletion of oxygen. This is followed by death and decay of all the aerobic organisms in the aqueous environment with the subsequent growth of anaerobic bacteria leading to the accumulation of toxins.

Exanthema An eruptive disease or fever.

Fatty acid An organic acid with a long aliphatic chain which may be saturated or unsaturated.

Fibrosis The formation of fibrous tissue which may be a response of tissue to injury resulting in increased amounts of collagen fibres.

Ficks Law At constant temperature the rate of diffusion of a substance across a cell membrane is proportional to the concentration gradient and the surface area.

First order process The rate of the process is proportional to the concentration of the substance.

First-pass metabolism Metabolism of a drug or other chemical during the absorption process. Typically occurs in the liver or gastrointestinal tract after oral dosing.

Food chain An imaginary chain of organisms existing in the environment in which each link of the chain feeds upon the one below and is eaten by the one above. At the bottom of the food chain are plants and bacteria, at the top are carnivores.

Free radical An atom or molecule which has an unpaired electron. They may be uncharged or charged depending on the numbers of electrons. Free radicals are usually chemically very reactive.

Genotoxic Toxic to the genetic material of an organism.

Glomerulus A functional unit of the vertebrate kidney consisting of a small bunch of capillaries projecting into a capsule (Bowmans capsule) which serves to collect the filtrate from the blood of those capillaries and direct it into the kidney tubule.

Glutathione (GSH) The tripeptide glutamyl-cysteinyl-glycine. Found in most tissues, especially the liver. Plays a major role in detoxication and cellular protection.

Glycoprotein A protein containing a carbohydrate moiety.

Good Laboratory Practice (GLP) A system of protocols (standard operating procedures) recommended to be followed so as to avoid the production of unreliable and erroneous data. Accurate record keeping and careful forethought in the design of the study are important aspects of GLP.

GSH/GSSG Reduced/oxidized glutathione.

Haemodialysis The process by which a foreign substance is removed from the blood of a poisoned patient by allowing it to diffuse across a semi-permeable membrane while the blood is pumped through a special machine.

Haemoglobinuria The presence of haemoglobin in the urine.

Haemolytic anaemia The pathological condition where red blood cells undergo uncontrolled destruction.

Haemoperfusion The process by which a foreign substance is removed from the blood of a poisoned patient by allowing it to be absorbed by activated charcoal or a resin while the blood is pumped through a special machine.

Haemorrhage The escape of blood from blood vessels.

Haemorrhagic necrosis Necrosis accompanied by bleeding.

Half-life The time taken for the concentration of a compound in a body fluid to decrease by half.

Hapten A molecule which becomes attached to a protein or other macromolecule and so renders it antigenic.

Henderson-Hasselbach equation $pH = pKa + \log A^-/HA$.

Histamine A mediator of inflammatory reactions in the body which may be part of an allergic reaction.

HLA type Histocompatability antigens on the surface of nucleated cells.

Hydrophobic/ hydrophilic A substance which repels/attracts water.

Hyperkinesis Hyperactivity.

Hypoglycaemia The physiological state where there is a low blood glucose concentration.

Hypoxia The physiological state where there is a low oxygen concentration in the tissues.

Idiosyncratic In toxicology this is an adverse reaction to a chemical which occurs in a single or small number of individuals as a result of an abnormality in that individual.

Immune complex A complex of antibody(ies) and antigen(s) which may lead to pathological consequences such as inflammation or blockage of a vessel.

Initiation The first stage in the multi-stage process of carcinogenesis in which there is thought to be a chemical reaction between the carcinogen and DNA.

Interferon A macromolecule produced by the body in response to a stimulus such as an infection.

Intraperitoneal/i.p. A route of administration of a compound to an animal by direct injection into the peritoneal cavity.

Irritation/ irritancy Direct injury to tissue such as the skin.

Ischaemia The condition where there is a reduced or blocked blood flow to a tissue which will lead to ischaemic tissue damage.

Isozyme/isoenzyme One of several forms of an enzyme where the different forms usually catalyze similar but distinct reactions.

Keratin A tough, fibrous protein found in the skin.
Killer lymphocyte A particular type of white blood cell involved in Type IV immunological reactions.

LD₅₀ The lethal dose of a compound for 50 per cent of the population of organisms exposed.
Lipid peroxidation Oxidative breakdown of lipids usually involving a free radical mechanism or active oxygen species and giving rise to reactive products which may be responsible for cellular damage.
Lipid solubility see lipophilicity.
Lipophilicity A term used to describe the ability of a substance to dissolve in, or associate with, fat and therefore living tissue. This usually applies to compounds which are non-ionized or non-polar or have a non-polar portion. Therefore high lipid solubility usually implies low water solubility.
Local toxicity Toxicity which affects only the site of application or exposure.

Macromolecule A very large molecule having a polymeric structure such as a protein or nucleic acid.
Macrophage Large phagocytic cells which are components of the reticuloendothelial system.
Maximally Tolerated Dose (MTD) The dose of a substance which causes no more than a 10 per cent weight decrease and does not cause death or any clinical signs of toxicity which would shorten the life span of an animal exposed for 90 days.
MEL Maximum Exposure Level; maximum level of occupational exposure of workers to a chemical; term used in UK.
Mesothelioma A rare form of cancer mainly affecting the pleura and caused exclusively by exposure to certain forms of asbestos.
Methaemoglobin/methaemoglobinaemia Oxidized haemoglobin/the syndrome in which a significant amount of the haemoglobin in the blood is oxidized.
Microflora/microfauna The bacteria and other organisms inhabiting the gastrointestinal tract.
Micronucleus test A test for mutagenicity (q.v.) using red blood cell stem cells from mice. The mice are exposed to the chemical and after a suitable time period the bone marrow examined for an increase in the number of micronuclei. These are chromosome fragments resulting from spindle or centromere dysfunction.
Microsomes/microsomal The subcellular fraction containing the fragments of the smooth endoplasmic reticulum (ER) after ultracentrifugation of a homogenate of the cell.
Mitochondria The intracellular organelle in which respiration and other important metabolic reactions take place.
Monooxygenase Enzyme system (such as cytochrome P450) involved in the oxidation of compounds.

Mutagen/mutagenic A substance/a property of a substance which causes some type of mutation in the genetic material of an organism exposed to it.

Mutagenesis Process in which a heritable change in DNA is produced.

Myocardium The middle and thickest layer of cardiac muscle in the heart wall.

NADH The coenzyme reduced nicotinamide adenine dinucleotide.

NADPH The coenzyme reduced nicotinamide adenine dinucleotide phosphate.

Narcosis Unconsciousness induced by exposure to a solvent or volatile liquid.

Necrosis Death of areas of tissue, usually surrounded by healthy tissue and sometimes caused by chemical exposure. As disinct from apoptosis, which is a limited event, necrosis also involves an inflammatory response and wider areas of tissue.

Nephritis Inflammation of the kidney.

Nephron The functional unit of the kidney which produces urine. It consists of a long tubule divided into sections in which reabsorption into the bloodstream of certain solutes filtered by the glomerulus from the blood takes place.

NOAEL No Observed Adverse Effect Level. The dose or exposure level at which no adverse effect is detected in the organism.

Occlusion Constriction or blockage as of a blood vessel.

Organelle A subcellular structure such as the mitochondrion or nucleus of a cell.

Osteomalacia Softening of the bones due to impaired mineralization.

Paresthesias Abnormal sensations such as tingling.

Partition coefficient Ratio of the solubility of a chemical in an aqueous solvent to that in a hydrophobic solvent. A high value indicates that a chemical is lipid-soluble (lipophilic).

Peripheral neuropathy Damage to nerves of the peripheral, rather than central, nervous system.

Peroxidases Enzymes which catalyze oxidation utilizing hydrogen peroxide. Found in many tissues including certain types of white blood cells (neutrophils).

Peroxisomal proliferators Chemicals which change the number and characteristics of peroxisomes (intracellular organelles which carry out oxidation of fatty acids).

Persistence When applied to a chemical substance meaning its ability to remain unchanged in the environment.

Pesticide An agent used to exterminate pests of various types. Includes insecticides, herbicides and fungicides.

Phago/pinocytosis The uptake of a solid substance (phago) or solution (pino) into a cell by invagination of the cell membrane eventually forming a vesicle inside the cell.

Pharmacodynamic Relating to the effects of drugs on living systems.

Phase 1 The term applied to the first stage of drug metabolism, commonly involving either oxidation, reduction or hydrolysis of the molecule.

Phase 2 The term applied to the second stage of drug metabolism usually involving conjugation of a functional group with a moiety available endogenously and conferring water solubility on the molecule.

Phase 3 Further metabolism of a metabolic product of a phase 2 reaction such as a glutathione conjugate.

Phenotype The expression of the genotype or genetic make-up of an organism.

Phocomelia The syndrome of having foreshortened arms and legs due to an adverse effect on the embryo such as caused by thalidomide.

Phospholipid A lipid in which one of the hydroxyl groups of glycerol or sphingosine is esterified with a phosphorylated alcohol.

pH Partition Theory This states that a foreign compound in the non-ionized state will pass across a cell membrane by passive diffusion down a concentration gradient.

Plasma Blood from which the cells have been removed by centrifugation but distinct from serum in which the blood is first allowed to clot.

Pneumonitis Inflammation of the lungs.

Polar A term used to describe a molecule which is charged or has a tendency to become polarized.

Polychlorinated biphenyls A group of compounds used industrially in which a biphenyl nucleus is substituted with various numbers of chlorine atoms.

Polypeptide A chain of amino acids joined by peptide bonds.

Portal The term applied to the venous circulation draining the tissues of the gastrointestinal tract into the liver.

Potentiation When the toxic effect of a compound is increased by a non-toxic compound.

PPAR Peroxisome proliferator activated receptor. Receptor involved in the induction of peroxisomal enzymes.

ppb Parts per billion.

ppm Parts per million. A measure of concentration of a substance in which the units of the substance are one millionth of the units of the solvent, e.g. μg per g.

Prescribed disease An industrial disease which is recognized as such for the purposes of compensation.

Promotion The second stage in the multi-stage process of carcinogenesis which must normally follow initiation in order for a tumour to develop.

Psychoactive drugs Drugs which produce behavioural changes.

Ptaquiloside Glucoside of a three-ring compound found naturally in bracken which yields a carcinogenic product.

Pulmonary oedema The accumulation of tissue fluid in the air spaces in the lungs.

Quantal response A response which is all-or-none rather than graded.

Rainout Removal of acids from the atmosphere by rain.

Raynauds phenomenon Changes in the blood supply to the fingers and toes which when caused by vinyl chloride results from degeneration of small blood vessels leading to occlusion of capillaries and arterioles.

Reaginic Relating to reagin, an antibody of the IgE type.

Renal elimination Excretion of a substance through the kidneys.

Rhinitis Inflammation of the mucous membranes of the nose.

Ribosomes The intracellular organelles attached to the endoplasmic reticulum which are involved with protein synthesis.

Risk 'Risk is a measure of the probability that an adverse effect will occur'. This may be absolute risk which is the excess risk due to exposure, or relative risk which is the ratio of risk in the exposed to the unexposed population.

Saturated A term applied to a molecule where all the bonds of the carbon atoms are utilized and there are no double or triple bonds.

Silicosis Damage to the lungs caused by exposure to substances such as silica or coal dust.

Singlet oxygen Oxygen in the singlet, excited state and therefore highly reactive.

Sinusoids Spaces filled with blood which in the liver are a continuation of the capillaries.

Skink Australian reptile.

Smog The term originally used to describe the combination *of smoke* and *fog* which is now termed reducing smog. Photochemical (oxidant) smog is the result of interaction between the pollution caused mainly by car exhausts and sunlight.

Steatosis Fatty infiltration in an organ or tissue.

Sub-chronic (28 or 90-day) An exposure of duration intermediate between acute and chronic.

Superoxide (O_2^-) The oxygen molecule with an extra and unpaired electron. It is thus a charged free radical.

Symport Membrane carrier system in which two substances are transported in the same direction.

Synergism/synergistic When toxic effect of a mixture is greater than the sum of the toxicities of the components.

Systemic toxicity Toxicity which affects a system in the organism other than and probably distant from the site of application or exposure.

TD_{50} The dose which is toxic to 50 per cent of the population of organisms exposed to the substance *or* a 50 per cent toxic response in a biological system exposed to the substance.

Teratogen/teratogenicity A substance/property of a substance causing abnormalities in the embryo or foetus when administered to the maternal organism.

Therapeutic index The ratio of ED_{50} to TD_{50}.

Thiol SH or sulphydryl group.

TLV Threshold Limit Value. Upper permissive limits of airborne concentrations of substances.

Tolerance When repeated administration of or dosing with a compound leads to a decrease in the potency in the biological activity of that compound.

Toxicodynamics Study of the effects of toxic substances on biological systems (e.g. interaction with receptors).

Toxicokinetics Study of the kinetics of toxic substances in biological systems (e..g. disposition).

Uniport Membrane carrier system in which one substance is transported in the one direction.

Unsaturated A term applied to molecules which contain double or triple carbon-carbon bonds.

Urticaria A vascular reaction of the skin marked by the appearance of weak and which may be caused by direct or indirect exposure to a toxic substance. Also known as hives.

Vascularized When relating to tissue meaning that it is supplied with vessels such as arteries or veins.

Vasculitis Inflammation of the vessels of the vascular system.

Vasodilation/vascular dilatation Dilation of blood vessels.

Veno-occlusive disease A particular type of liver damage where the blood vessels and sinusoids of the liver are damaged so that new vessels grow.

Volume of distribution (V_D) The volume of body fluid in which a compound is apparently distributed when administered to an animal.

Washout Removal of acids from clouds by rain.

Zero order process The rate of the process is independent of the concentration of the substance.

Index